A HOUSE HUSBANDS' GUIDE

A HOUSE HUSBANDS' GUIDE

Cooking for your pregnant partner

AARON HARVIE

NH
NEW
HOLLAND

For Natalie and Isabella

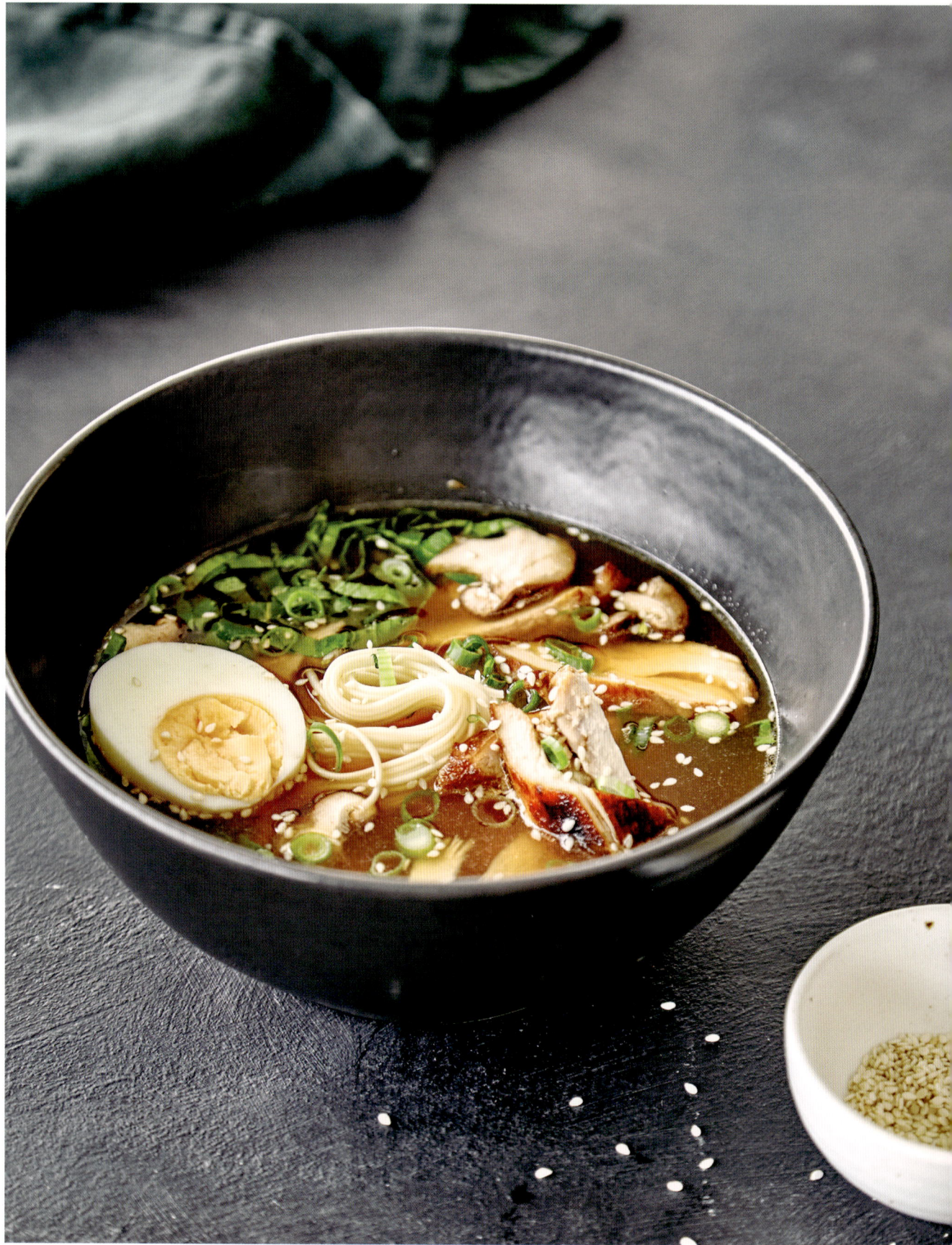

CONTENTS

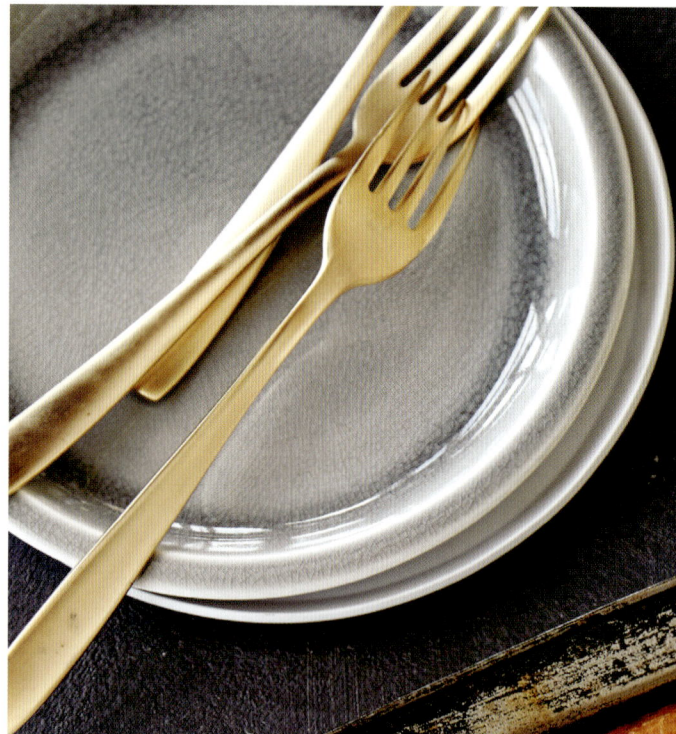

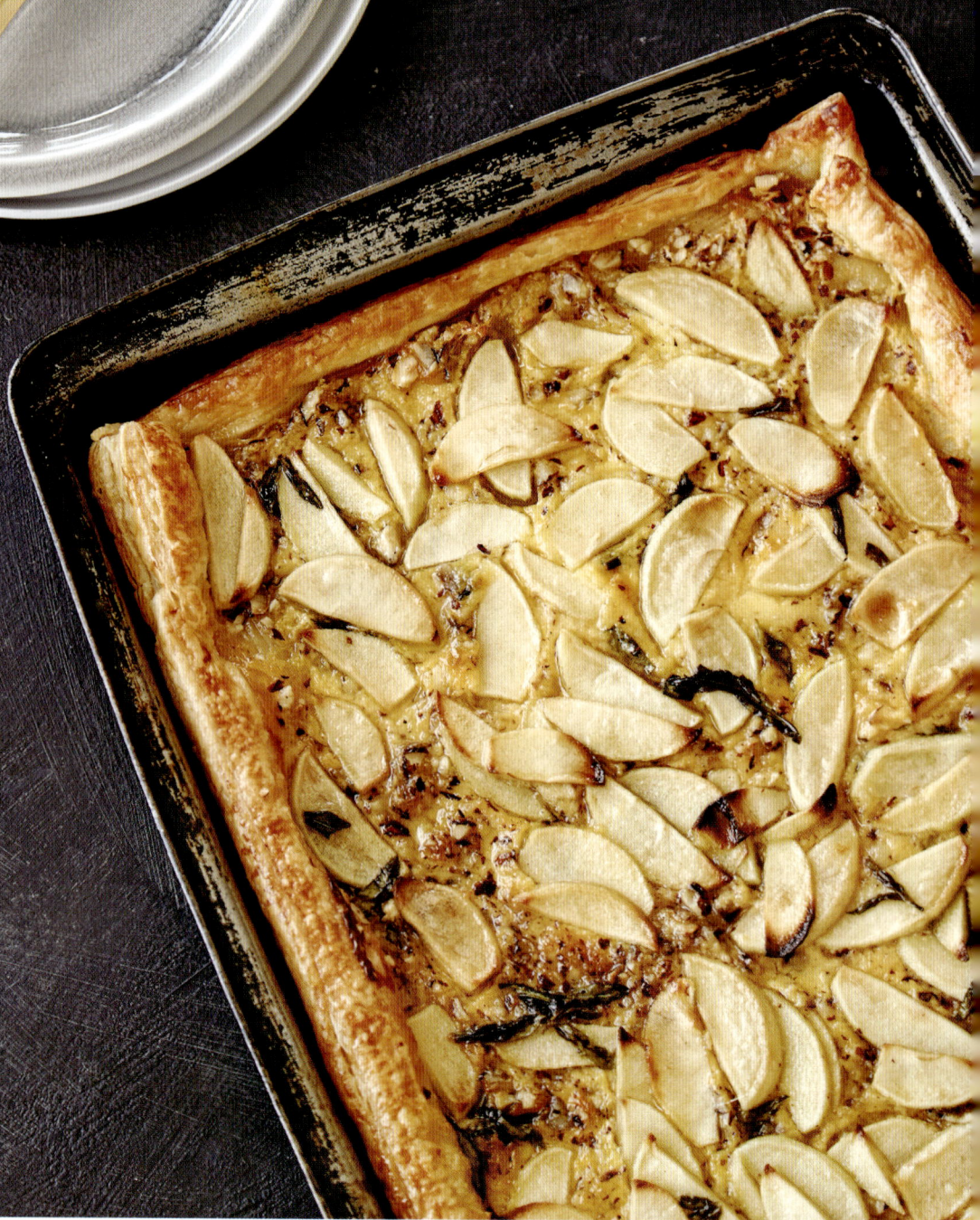

INTRODUCTION

Pregnancy cooking: the last time in a long time you can feed a meal to your child without it coating the walls.

They say you fall in love the moment you see your newborn baby for the first time. Now, I'd like to say that was true, but in my case if I'm being totally honest, it didn't quite happen like that.

The first emotion I felt was fear. Fear that my newborn daughter was going to be alright after a traumatic entrance into the world, fear that my wife wouldn't recover after complications with her delivery and fear that I would be able to measure up and be the best father I could possibly be for this wrinkled, purple mess that was screaming in the delivery room in front of me. The fact that this tiny little baby was so totally and utterly helpless only served to fuel my anxiety which soon gripped my chest and squeezed it tight like a vice, making it impossible to breath. Then instinctively my daughter, who was only a couple of minutes old, reached out and took a hold of the index finger of my left hand squeezing it tightly. I had never known a calm like that before and all at once the fear washed away, knowing she was here with me now and forever apart of my life. And from that moment onwards I was done, I was hers totally and completely.

I was in love.

Regardless of whether you're expecting your first bundle of joy, welcoming an unplanned matching set or adding to an ongoing series you've been collecting for some time, you will no doubt be preparing for the monumental change that is about to come crashing down over you like a tsunami, forever washing away the life that you once knew. And the first of these many, many changes is the actual pregnancy itself.

It's easy to feel a little removed and alienated at the start of your partner's pregnancy. While they begin to go through this incredible physical metamorphosis nurturing an unborn child, things for you remain relatively unchanged and your involvement can sometimes feel limited to simply being there and offering support. But there is a way to get more involved and make a major contribution to your partner's pregnancy and give your baby the best possible start in life. Food

By simply making an effort, getting into the kitchen and cooking the meals, you can support your partner and also help ensure your baby gets the nutrition they need at the same time. And by some amazing twist of fate or incredible biological coincidence, being acknowledged for simply making an effort is one of the things we, as men, love most of all. In fact, as minimal as that effort may be sometimes, the fact that we have made one at all is a cause for celebration as far as we're concerned.

The nutritional needs of an expectant mother can be a little intimidating if you are not experienced in the kitchen and it's natural to feel a little unsure of what you should be cooking. Unfortunately for any expectant mother, especially those with a slightly adventurous palette, the dietary intake required means meals can quickly become repetitive, bland and very restrictive. Add raging hormones, morning sickness, swollen feet and an ever-expanding belly to the mix and you've got yourself one very unhappy partner!

Like it or not, there are many culinary sins that need to be committed in the name of food safety during the three trimesters of pregnancy to ensure you are cooking safely for your partner and unborn baby. If you peruse the dietary restrictions and food safety advice provided by your medical practitioner, it can be downright depressing when you realise just how many things need to be given up or changed dramatically to be considered safe. Eggs can only be served hard-boiled, red meat needs to be cooked through and served well-done (something that still makes me wake up screaming in the middle of the night), you can't eat sashimi or sushi, cold-cured meats are a no-go as well as soft cheeses, bean sprouts, home-made mayonnaise and soft serve ice-cream. Even the stuffing from a roast turkey or chicken during the festive season is off the menu.

What's worse is when you finally figure out what's okay to eat, you soon discover there is also a never-ending list of dos and don'ts you need to be aware of when it comes to leftovers and food temperatures. And after all of this, if you're the kind of person who believes in solidarity and decide you are going to eat the same diet as your partner during the pregnancy, you will soon realise that not only will you will have to endure this culinary crime spree, you'll have to do it while you're totally sober.

For nine long months.

So this book is designed to be a bit of a lifeline, a helping hand for those of you out there who are looking to get involved and cook some different dishes for your partner. It's not a nutritional eating plan, nor does it contain some revolutionary diet for your partner to follow—the experts at the hospital and your doctor already have that covered. Instead, what you'll find inside this book are recipes, hints and tips to help you in the kitchen, regardless of your skill level.

WHAT THE HECK IS FOLATE?

A fool's guide to what your partner can and can't eat

There are many terms that are being bandied about when you find out your partner is pregnant and straight off the bat it feels as if you are expected to know what doctors and health care professionals are talking about. Lactating, Mastitis, Braxton Hicks contractions, folate, uterus, amniotic fluid, ectopic pregnancy, Nuchal Translucency Test. I mean, sure, I heard some of these terms before but what they meant and more importantly how they were applicable to our situation left me sitting in the doctor's office scratching my head with my eyes glazed over, just like when I was back in school.

Was there really such a thing as a lactation consultant or was this something made up, like the Easter Bunny?

What was this 'show' everybody kept talking about and should we invite our family and friends along to see it when it happened?

Was the person who names medical procedures having a bad day and really over their job when they came up with the term vacuum extraction?

The reality of the situation is that if you take the time to read the information you receive from your doctor or health care provider, all the questions you have regarding your partner's pregnancy are pretty much covered and anything else you want to know you simply just have to ask the question. Remember you're not a fool for asking a question, even if you think it's stupid. You're a fool for not asking the question and going along like you know the answer.

When it comes to food, if you and your partner normally eat a balanced and sensible diet prior to pregnancy then the changes you have to make to follow the prescribed dietary guidelines are not all that dramatic.

And if you don't, well, you may be in for a bit of a shock.

Lots of leafy greens, fruit and vegetables, breads, cereals, rice and pasta, most dairy (or dairy alternatives), lean meats, eggs, poultry and fish (if you eat meat) plus plenty of water is in essence all you really need (aside from following a few food safety guidelines). If you are unsure about whether or not your partner should eat something, it's better to err on the side of caution until you have checked it's okay.

Detailed eating plans, as well as dietary advice, should come from your medical practitioner. The following are some common terms you may hear, as well as a couple of tips and tricks for preparing food safely and still making it taste great.

FOLATE

Folate and folic acid are two words that pop up again and again and you will become very familiar with them while looking at the dietary requirements of your baby's early development.

Simply put, folates and folic acid can help prevent neural tube birth abnormalities.

You can find folates in lots of things including leafy greens and broccoli as well as chickpeas, nuts, dried beans and fruits. Many countries now also add folic acid to breads, breakfast cereals and juices so make sure you check on the nutrition information panel when you're in the supermarket.

IRON

A developing baby needs iron and your baby is going to draw it from its mother faster than a toddler is going to draw on a freshly painted white wall with a crayon. Or couch. Or table. Or priceless family heirloom. (Anyway you get the idea, pretty quickly.)

So, to make sure your partner gets enough iron you should make sure they eat foods that are high in Vitamin C (helps iron absorption), reduce caffeine consumption (reduces iron absorption) and eat a sufficient amount of lean red meat, chicken or fish, eggs, legumes or green vegies like spinach, Asian greens, peas or broccoli.

CALCIUM

Here's a no brainer: we all need calcium in our diet. For pregnant women however, it's a must as it helps the development of baby's teeth and bones. If your partner doesn't have enough calcium in their diet the baby is going to draw it straight from the mother, so to avoid the risk of brittle bones, fractures or osteoporosis later in life, make sure there's plenty of calcium in your diet. Consuming milk, yoghurt and hard cheese is the easiest way to make sure you are getting enough. If you don't do dairy you'll be happy to know that most Asian greens, broccoli, almonds and tinned fish will also get you over the line.

IODINE

There are quite a few countries in the world now where the population is experiencing varying levels of iodine deficiency, which in babies can be the cause of stunted growth and intellectual disabilities. Many of these countries, including Australia, have now embarked on an iodine fortification program in commercially sold bread to combat the issue. Iodine can be found naturally in seafood and seaweed, as well as sea salt and iodised table salt.

Fish and other seafood is something you want to keep in your partner's diet but it is important to note that while it is high in protein and omega-3 fatty acids, they can contain mercury which can cause developmental issues in babies. Doctors recommend 2–3 serves of fish a week for all fish, except for deep sea perch and catfish which should not be consumed more than once a week, with no other fish on the menu, and large predatory fish, shark (flake), swordfish, rays, barramundi and ling, which should not be consumed more than once a fortnight with no other fish on the menu.

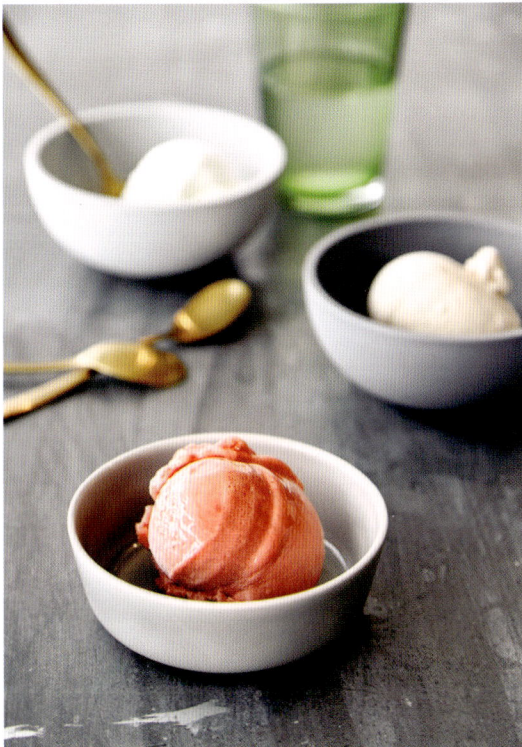

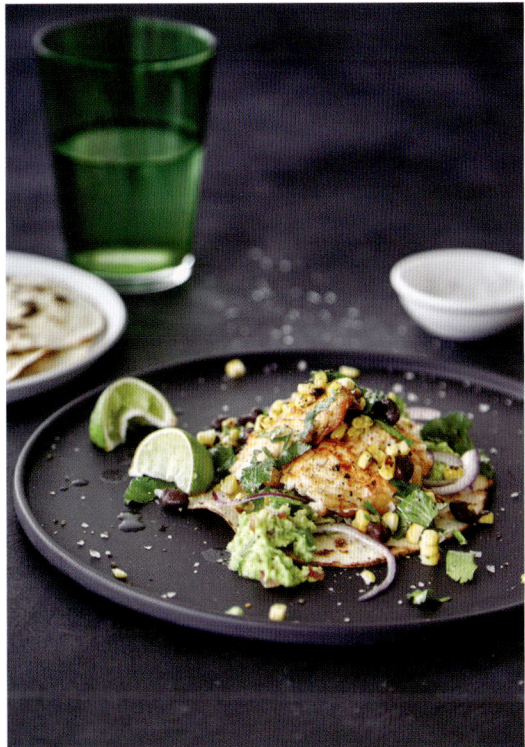

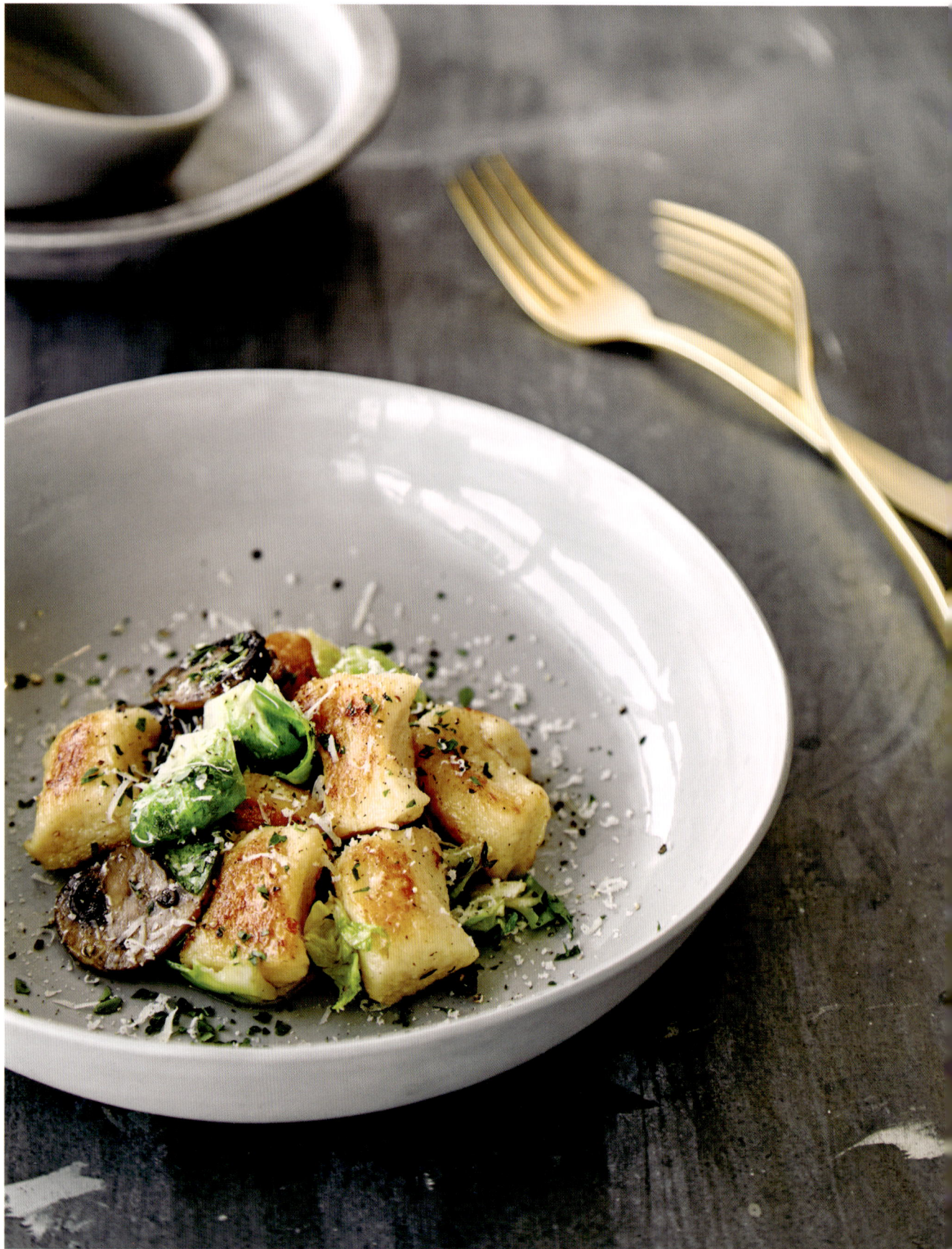

CHEATS, TRICKS & A COUPLE OF TIPS

SHAKES... EVERYTHING YOU NEED IN ONE QUICK DRINK

I will never forget the look of horror in my wife's eyes when she realised just how much she had to consume, day in and day out to follow the nutritional guidelines recommended by our doctor. Four to six servings of breads and cereals, five to six servings of vegetables, four servings of fruit, one and a half servings of protein and two servings of calcium.

Every. Single. Day.

Of course, pregnant women take supplements to ensure that most of these nutritional needs are met but the amount of food they need to consume is a lot. Throw in morning sickness, extreme fatigue, aches and pains and the fact that they have a person growing inside of them and this can be a daunting proposition.

My wife did not have that much trouble consuming the recommended daily intake of food at the start of her pregnancy and, aside from combating nausea, it didn't seem like too much of a challenge. However, the second and especially the third trimester is when things tend to get a little tricky because as the child continues to grow larger and larger, a woman's organs need to shift dramatically to accommodate this change. By the third trimester, a pregnant mother's liver and lungs have been repositioned, her intestines and bladder are way over yonder and her stomach has been squeezed and cramped so it's much harder for her to consume the same amount of food.

I found shakes and homemade juices for either breakfast or lunch (or in between meals as a snack to avoid bloating) a great way to fulfil the dietary requirements because I could jam together many of the things she needed into one glass.

MAKE EATING AT HOME AS FUN AS EATING OUT

One of the important rules to make meat products safe to consume for our pregnant partners is to cook them through to well done so as to minimise the chance of food poisoning and exposure to harmful bacteria. For

15

some it's no big deal to eat well-done meat and eggs while for others the thought of nine months without a rare steak, cold-cured meats, duck liver pâté or a slightly runny egg is enough to send them screaming down the halls. in need of years of counselling.

The truth is that some of the food safety requirements and dietary limitations can start to feel more than a little restrictive by the second trimester and your partner may start wearing a brave face of disappointment more often than not, especially when you dine out.

Unfortunately, there is no getting around the fundamental laws of science but you can get some of your partners favourite dishes back on the menu with a little creative thinking. One of the things my wife craved most was a Vietnamese sandwich better known in the western world as a Bánh mì. Now this innocent (and downright delicious) sandwich was off limits because it contained pâté and the meat and salad were stored in a refrigerated sandwich bar, which can be a haven for certain food-borne nasties. But by simply cooking the chicken at home and serving it hot, making the salads fresh and substituting mushroom for liver in the pâté it was easy to get this dish back on the menu and restore a smile to my wife's face.

The same creative thinking can be applied to most dishes and while they may not taste exactly the same, making that much of an effort has got to make your partner happy and in turn make you look good. And in the end, that should be reason enough.

LIFE IS SO MUCH EASIER WITH ASIAN GREENS ON THE MENU

You will notice throughout this book I have included many recipes that have their origins in Asia. There are several reasons for this. First, there is an extraordinary amount of extremely tasty dishes that originate from this region that feature a lot of the vegetables that pregnant women need to eat. Second, in the time-poor state that many of us find ourselves in, most of these dishes are easy to cook and unlike some other cuisines, the use of pre-made sauces and stocks is not only acceptable, it's expected.

As a whole, Asian greens are versatile to cook with and are great in everything from soups to stir-fries. They come in endless varieties like bok choy (pak choy), choy sum (Chinese flowering cabbage), gai choy (Chinese mustard greens), gai larn (Chinese broccoli), kangkong (water spinach), mizuna and wong bok (Chinese cabbage), to name but a few. They are packed to the brim with those prized folates, as well as being low in calories, high in fibre and containing iron, calcium and vitamin C among a host of other beneficial goodies your partner needs.

The great thing about Asian greens is the simplicity and speed of their preparation— even if you're busy, a healthy meal can be made in minutes. Don't believe me? Well simply turn on your rice cooker and while it's working its magic, toss some bok choy in a wok with some ginger, garlic and oyster sauce. Dinner is served literally in the time it takes to make rice in a rice cooker.

EGGS

To me, the egg is the most versatile, satisfying and interesting food we cook with. Unlike many ingredients, it is used in both savoury and sweet cooking, it is acceptable to be served for breakfast, lunch or dinner and we can use almost any method concocted by humankind to prepare them.

So when the perfectly poached, custardy, soft-boiled, velvety saucy or sunny side fried versions of the egg are suddenly off the menu because of our selfish and downright nauseating friend salmonella, it gets me a little perturbed. Don't get me wrong, I am happy to eat the hard-boiled kind but it's easy to get pretty sick of them pretty quickly.

Our friend the humble egg is a great source of protein, iron, calcium as well as vitamin A and folate so it is important to keep them in our partner's diet, so the question remains, what can I do with eggs if they must be fully cooked through?

The simplest methods are to serve them hard-boiled, scrambled or in omelettes but I found the best way to deal with this dilemma was simply conceal them in other ingredients and preparations. You can add a hard-boiled egg to a ramen, or make a frittata or a quiche, chop them up with fried sourdough, white beans and spinach in a salad or simply conceal them in a sandwich mixed with store-bought mayonnaise. And who knows, get creative enough and you may make something so good that you start to enjoy your eggs hard-boiled from now on (but you'd have to get pretty darn creative if you ask me).

The one huge advantage that eggs have over a lot of other foods is in their preparation. If you boil them, you can't smell them cooking. So if your partner is feeling green around the gills and the smell of food is turning her stomach, having a little war chest of boiled eggs can prove very useful.

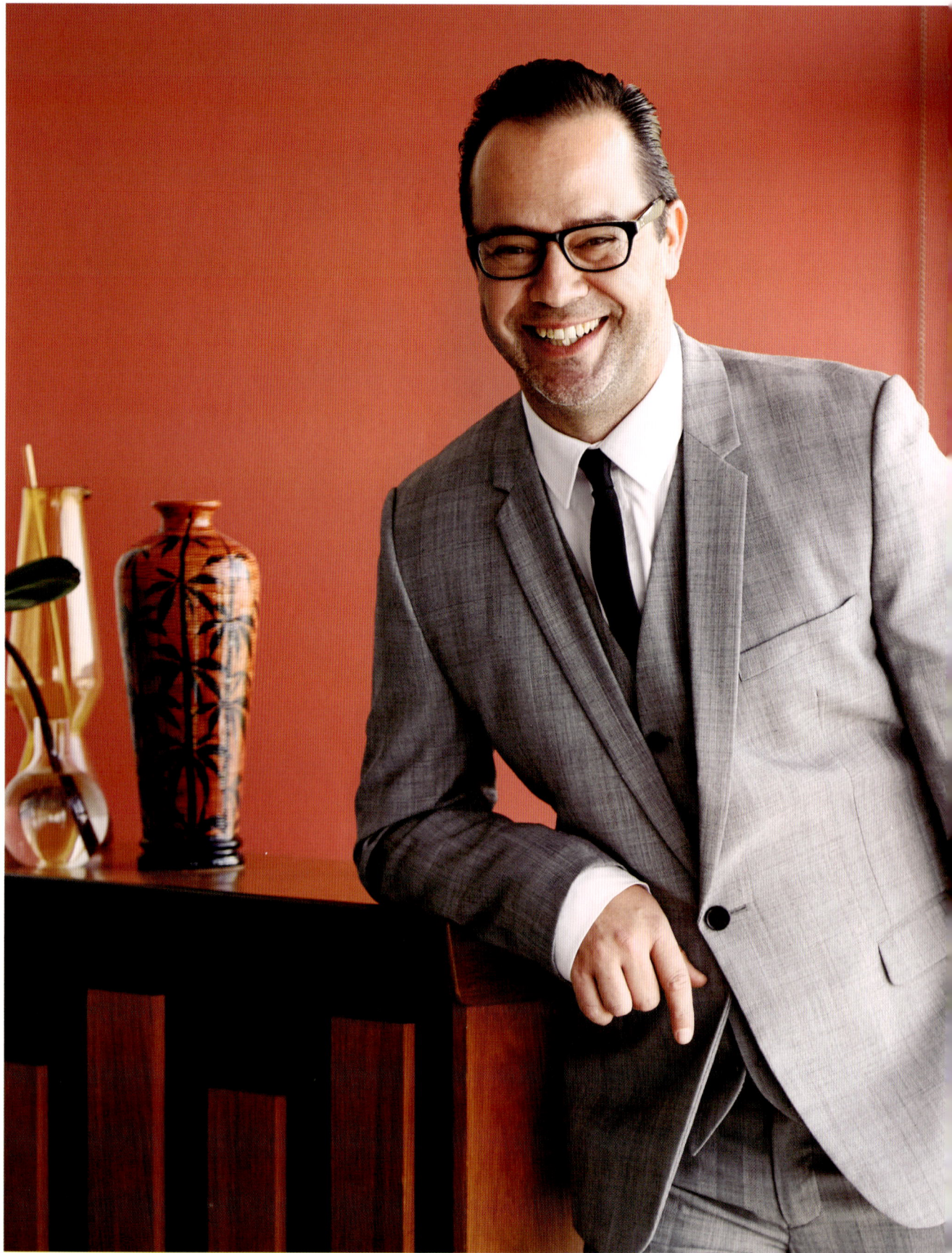

THE THREE SECOND RULE

Kitchen hygiene, prep methods, food borne nasties
and how to avoid them

Most of these rules and kitchen tips go without saying. I mean, we all use the kitchen every day so this section should really be a bit of a no-brainer. But as food poisoning and bacterial contamination can be especially serious during pregnancy, let's just pretend we know nothing and go over the basics one more time.

WASH YOUR HANDS
Anti-bacterial soap (or whatever you are comfortable with) near the kitchen sink is a must. And gentlemen, don't just rinse your hands, wash them properly: fingers, fingernails, palms and thumbs. It should take a minimum of 10 seconds.

KEEP THE KITCHEN CLEAN
While this may not make much sense, you will actually spend less time in the kitchen and become much more efficient if you clean as you go and keep your kitchen uncluttered as you cook. Before each session in the kitchen, wipe down all your benches, make sure you have a tea-towel handy when you're cooking, keep a bowl on the kitchen bench for scraps (saves you running to and touching the bin all the time), wash dishes and utensils as you go, put food away after it's been used, make sure you use separate cutting boards and wash your knives when preparing both meat and vegetables.

IF IT FALLS ON THE FLOOR IT GOES IN THE BIN
Think of all the places you walk around while wearing your shoes. Bathroom floors. Trains. Gutters. Stepping

in something in the park. Now think of dropping food on the same surface your shoes have been on. Not too pretty. The truth is that if you drop something on the kitchen floor, bacteria, including Salmonella and E. coli, can contaminate it instantly. So err on the side of caution, toss it in the bin and start again.

WASH FRUIT, VEGETABLES AND SALAD STUFFS
A rinse under the tap can remove pesticides, chemical residue and dirt which can harbour all kinds of micro-nasties including Toxoplasmosis, Salmonella and E. coli.

KEEP PETS OUT OF THE KITCHEN
Again, really shouldn't have to be said but pets have no place where food you are going to eat is prepared. While we all love our pets we wouldn't want to see a dog digging around for scraps in the kitchen of our favourite pizza place or a cat cleaning itself on the prep bench at a fine dining restaurant. If your dog's bowl is normally kept in the kitchen it's a good idea to keep them somewhere else. If you cat likes to walk on the kitchen benches, be vigilante and wipe them down with an antibacterial wipe before cooking.

STORE RAW OR PERISHABLE INGREDIENTS IN THE FRIDGE
We are not reinventing the wheel with this one. If it's perishable it goes in the fridge or the freezer. When you're shopping, especially in summer, it's not a bad idea to take a cool bag to the supermarket with you.

DEFROST FOOD IN THE FRIDGE
This takes a little longer and requires a bit of forethought and planning but to ensure raw food is not being contaminated it is best to place it in a bowl (you don't want frozen food juices dripping in the fridge) and defrost in the fridge. Bacteria can multiply and create toxins at temperatures between 5˚C (41˚F) and 60˚C (140˚F) but they really go to town on each other between 21˚C (70˚F) and 47˚C (117˚F), which makes a warm day like a party at Studio 54 for these little buggers.

IF YOU HAVE GASTRO, EAT OUT
No, this is not some play on molecular gastronomy or a gastro-pub, I'm talking about good old-fashioned gastroenteritis. If you have any of the symptoms, it's a good idea to hang up the apron and take a couple of nights off as it is very easy to pass this on to your partner if you are cooking or even handling food.

DON'T EAT FOOD PAST IT'S USE BY DATE
Enough said.

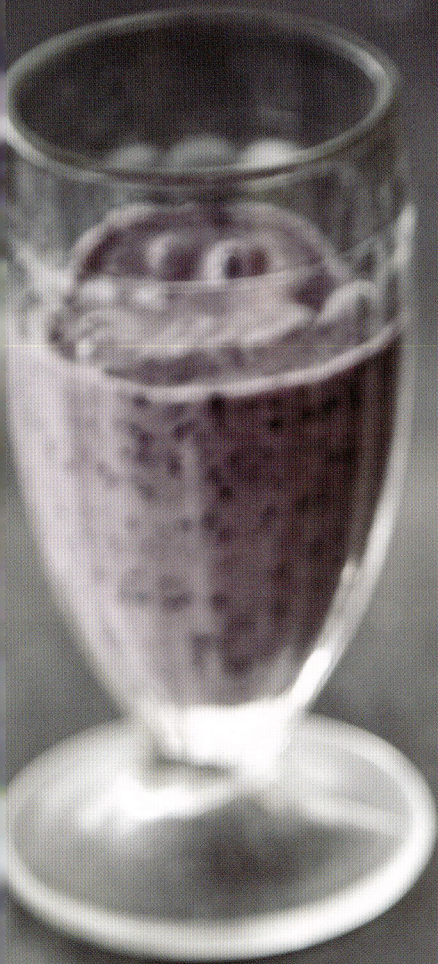

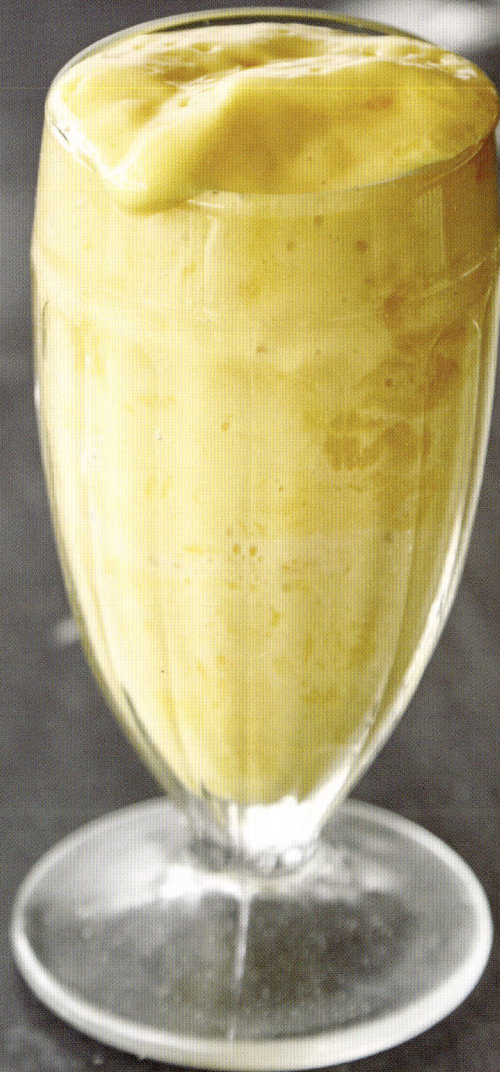

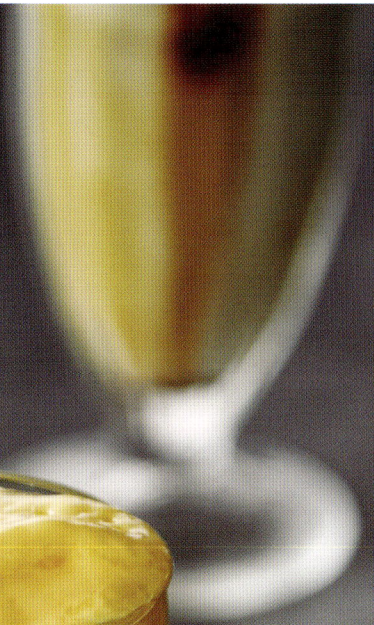

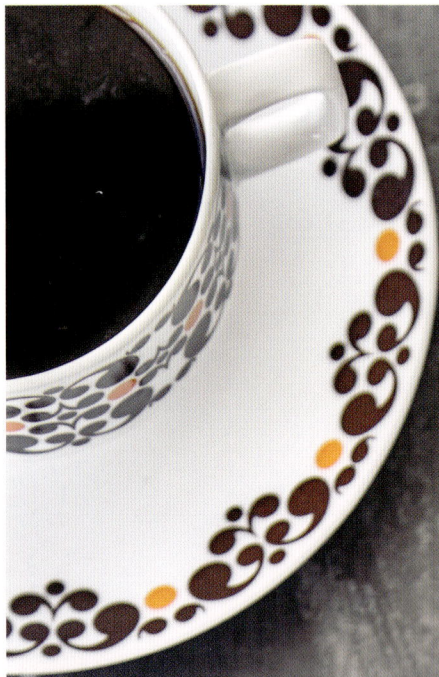

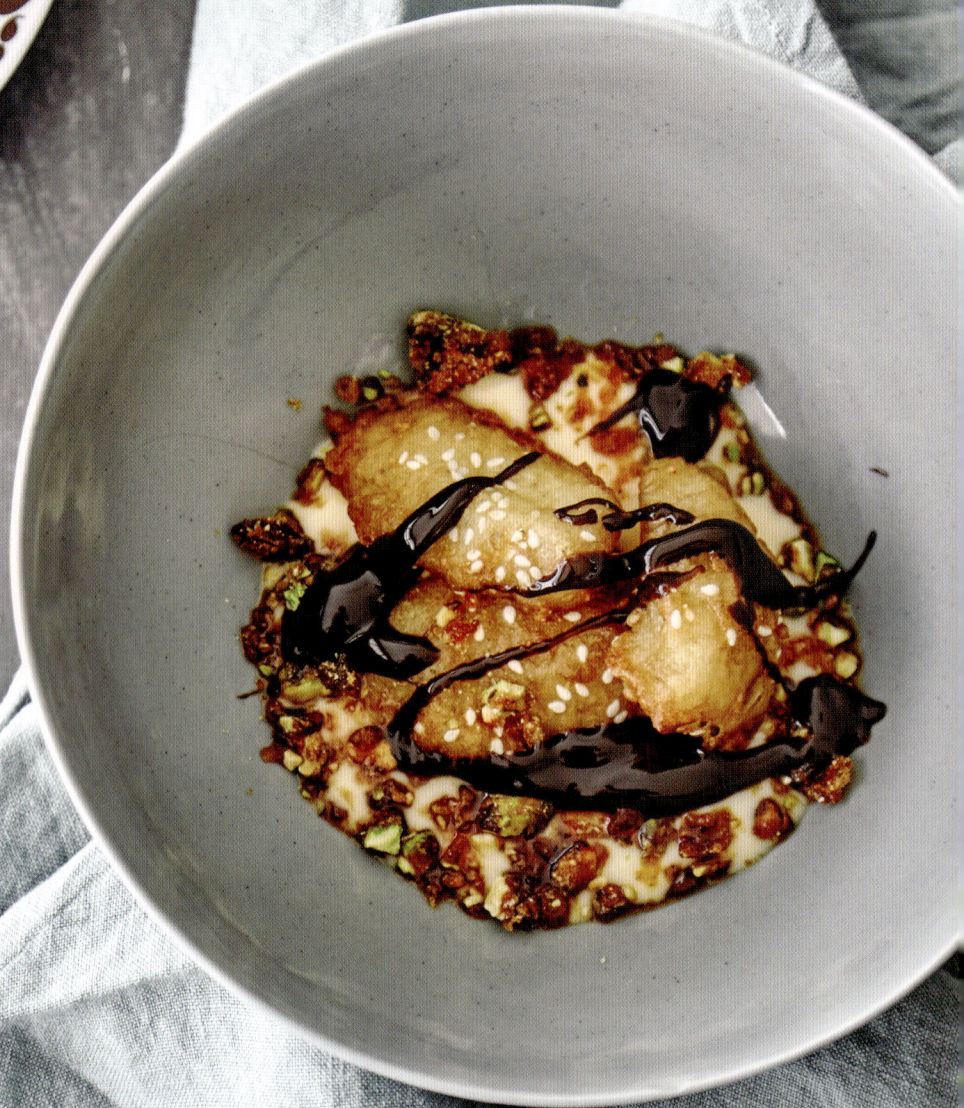

WHAT'S ON THE MENU & WHAT'S OFF

The good, and not-so-good stuff.

MEATS, POULTRY & FISH

What's Off?

× Forget about anything raw
× No cold processed meats (salami, prosciutto, etc.)
× No cold chicken, meat or seafood and no store-bought sushi
× No pâté or store-bought meat spreads

What's On?

× Processed meats (salami, prosciutto etc.) are okay if they have been heated to 75°C (167°F) and consumed hot Red meat must be cooked to 71°C (160°F) and consumed hot
× Poultry must be cooked to 74°C (165°F) and consumed hot
× Seafood must be cooked to 63°C (145°F) and consumed hot

To be on the safe side, cook until there is no pink in a steak, the juices run clear in poultry and for seafood, the meat is not translucent

EGGS

What's Off?

× No raw eggs, which means no homemade mayonnaise, mousse, meringue or re-enacting the training scene from Rocky
× No homemade ice-cream, sabayon, hollandaise or anything where eggs are not heated to 71°C (160°F)
× No soft serve ice cream or fried ice-cream

What's On?

- ˣ Eggs must be cooked through to well-done or hard-boiled—71˚C (160˚F)
- ˣ Store-bought custard can be eaten cold on the day and the next day must be heated to 60˚C (140˚F)
- ˣ Commercial mayonnaise and aïoli
- ˣ Commercial ice-cream

DAIRY

What's Off?

- ˣ No soft and semi-soft cheeses, which I'm afraid to say includes no ricotta, brie, camembert, feta, neufchâtel, havarti, munster-géromé, Port Salut, bleu de Laqueuille, crème fraîche, gorgonzola, mascarpone and a myriad of other gooey gastronomical godsends, unless they have been heated to 75˚C (167˚F) and consumed hot
- ˣ No unpasteurised dairy products

What's On?

- ˣ Processed cheeses like cream cheese and cottage cheese can be consumed but must be eaten within 2 days of opening
- ˣ Hard cheeses, such as cheddar, colby, gouda, parmesan, pecorino, Swiss, tasty, are good to go but check particular types before consuming.
- ˣ Soft cheeses like bocconcini, mozzarella and provolone are safe if bought pre-packaged and not from the deli counter but always check particular types before consuming.
- ˣ Milk, cream, yoghurt, etc. (but they MUST be pasteurised).

VEGIES & FRUIT

What's Off?

- ˣ No pre-packaged salads or stuff from sandwich bars and salad bars.
- ˣ No sprouts unless cooked to 75˚C (167˚F) and consumed hot.

What's On?

- ˣ Almost everything else but thoroughly wash fruit and veg before eating.

REHEATING & LEFTOVERS

As a rule, leftovers last a day in the fridge. Anything that is going to be saved as a leftover *must* be stored in the fridge and not left out for longer than 2 hours. All leftovers must be reheated so they are steaming hot at a minimum of 60°C (140°F).

FOOD POISONING, HARMFUL BACTERIA & COMMON SENSE

Foodborne illnesses are of major concern during a pregnancy. Not only because expectant mothers are much more susceptible due to changes in their immune system but also because harmful bacteria can cross through the placenta to the unborn child, whose immune system is way too underdeveloped to fight it. This can lead to serious problems including miscarriage or premature delivery and, in extreme cases, even death. The consequences and repercussions associated with foodborne nasties are too great to ignore and although the chance of contracting them and experiencing adverse complications are relatively low, they are easy to avoid. When you think about it, a little inconvenience; is not much of a price to pay for giving your child the best chance to have a healthy start in life.

LISTERIA

Listeria is a type of bacteria commonly found in soil that can cause an infection called listeriosis. This bacterium is of particular concern because unlike other foodborne pathogens, it can grow in refrigerated temperatures and once a food preparation factory is infected it can be very difficult to get rid of (which is why a lot of pre-packaged salads are on the naughty list). Symptoms can range from nothing at all to feeling like you have the flu in adults but the infection can be fatal for unborn babies. Therefore, it is important that anyone thinking they may have eaten contaminated food should present themselves to their healthcare professional immediately for testing.

   While listeriosis infection is severe, the good news is that it's rare, but pregnant women should be aware that soft and semi-soft cheeses, cold-pressed meats, cold cooked chicken, pre-packaged salads, fruit and vegetables, pâté, soft serve ice cream and raw seafood all have a higher risk of containing the bacteria.

SALMONELLA

Salmonella is a type of bacteria that can cause an infection called salmonellosis. It is mainly spread by eating undercooked, contaminated food, or coming into contact with a person infected with the bacteria who has not washed their hands properly. It can cause a range of symptoms including headache, fever, diarrhoea and vomiting in the mother while causing severe complications or even death in unborn babies if the bacteria manages to cross the placenta.

   Salmonella can be avoided by ensuring that all food is thoroughly cooked through and served hot. Food should never be consumed if it is raw or undercooked. Anyone preparing food should practice good hygiene and wash hands properly (including under the fingernails). All food preparation areas and equipment should be cleaned after each use and all food should be washed before preparation and stored below 5°C (41°F).

If you are the cook and you are suffering from a tad of intestinal distress (that's diarrhoea, between you and me) you should not cook, handle or prepare food for your partner until 48 hours after it has stopped. No exceptions.

TOXOPLASMOSIS

Toxoplasmosis is a parasitic disease caused by the ingestion of raw or undercooked meat containing cysts, cat faeces, contaminated soil or drinking untreated water (which includes tap water in developing nations). Most of the time it is non-symptomatic or causes mild flu-like symptoms but in congenital toxoplasmosis it can cause severe complications, miscarriage or even death to the unborn child.

You can take steps to avoid toxoplasmosis by ensuring you don't eat raw or undercooked meat (see the pattern forming here), unpasteurised dairy and unwashed fruit and vegies. Wash your hands after touching pets, especially cats, wear gloves while digging in the garden, don't drink water from a lake, river or overseas tap water and above anything else, get someone else to change the kitty litter.

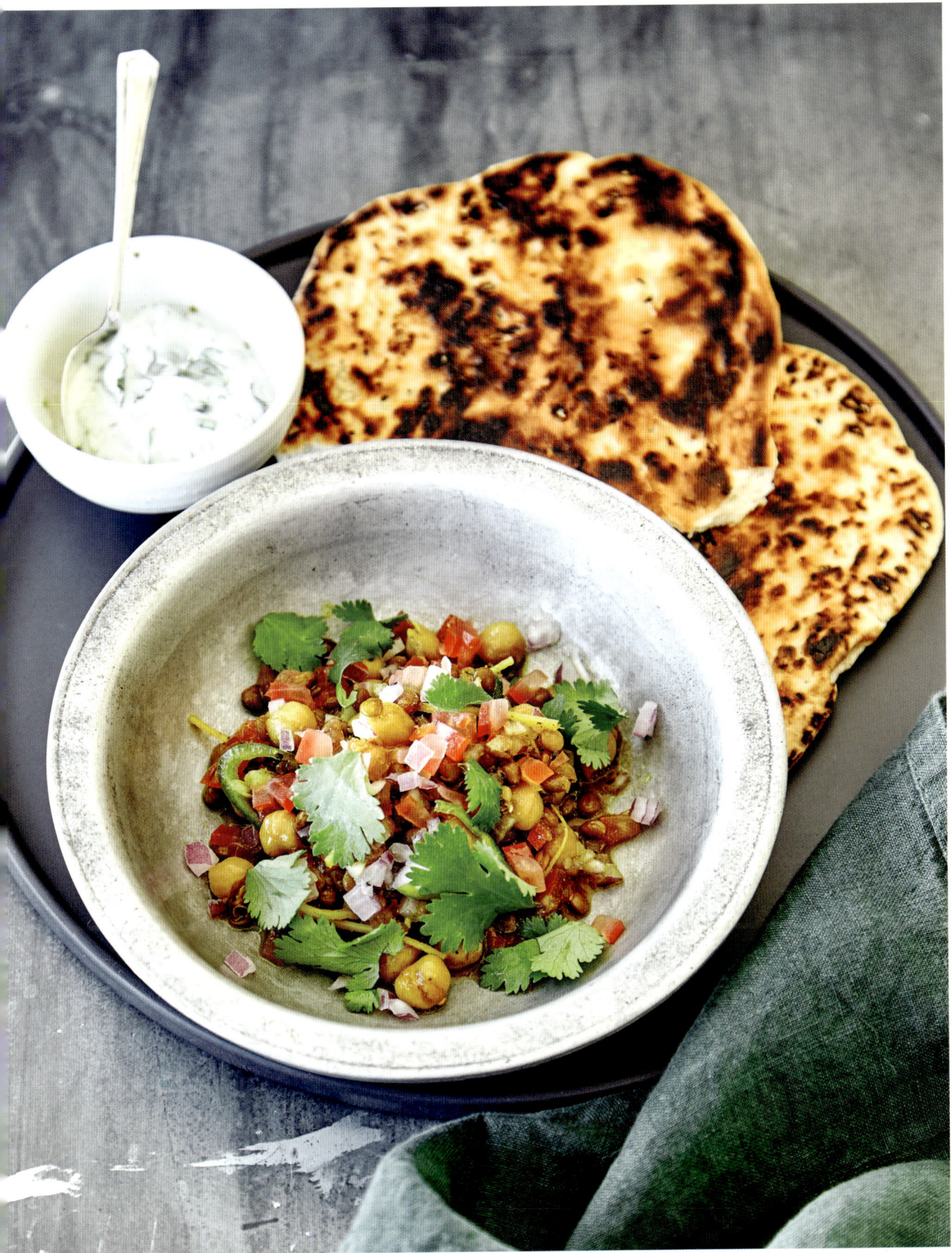

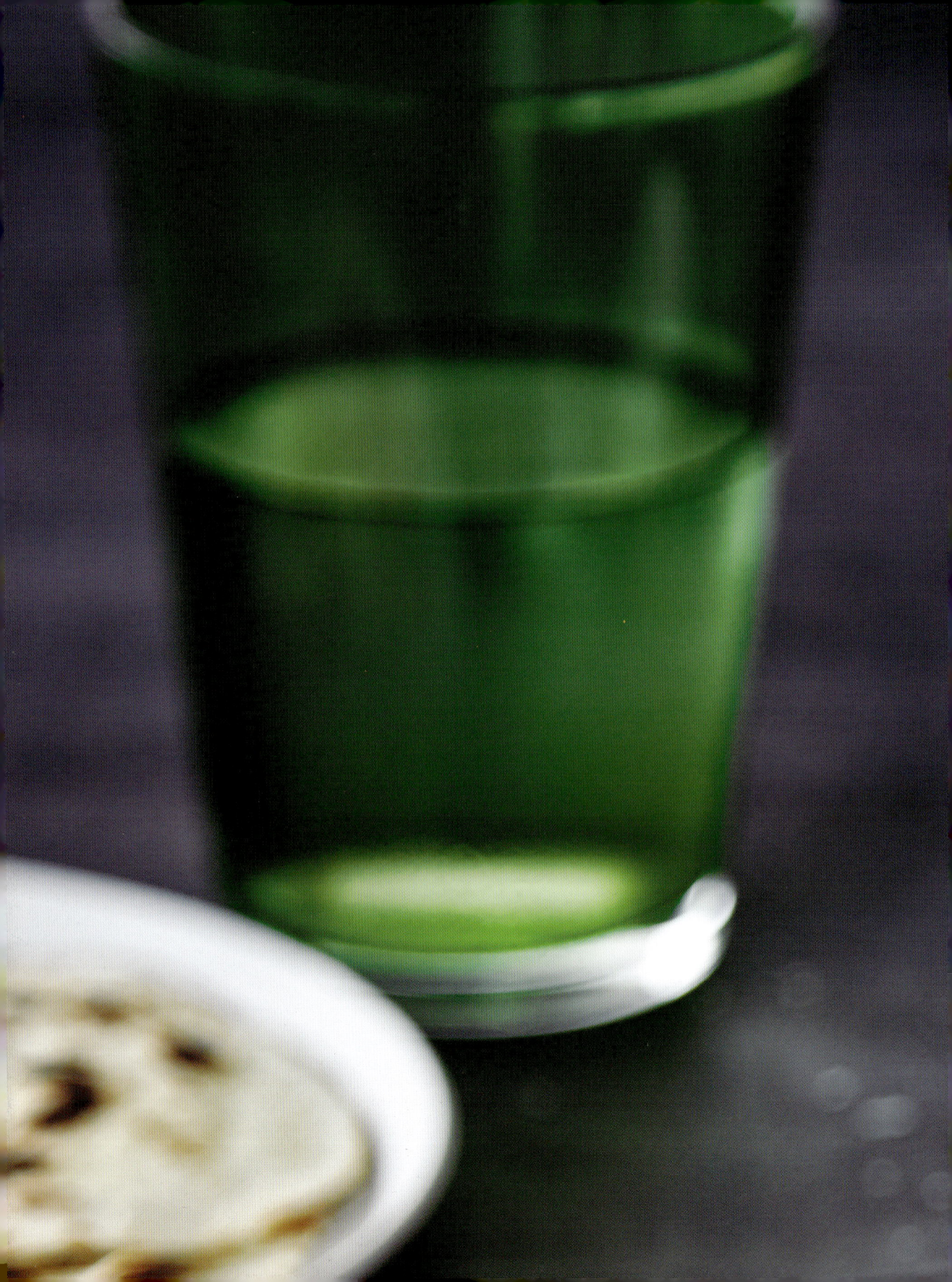

BASICS

The stuff you need in the kitchen

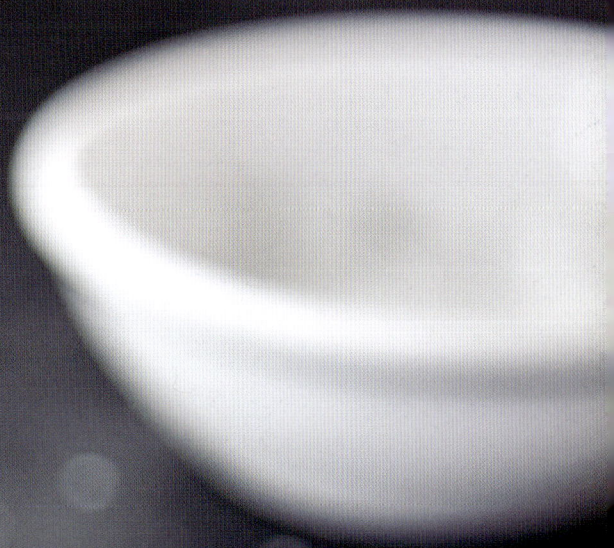

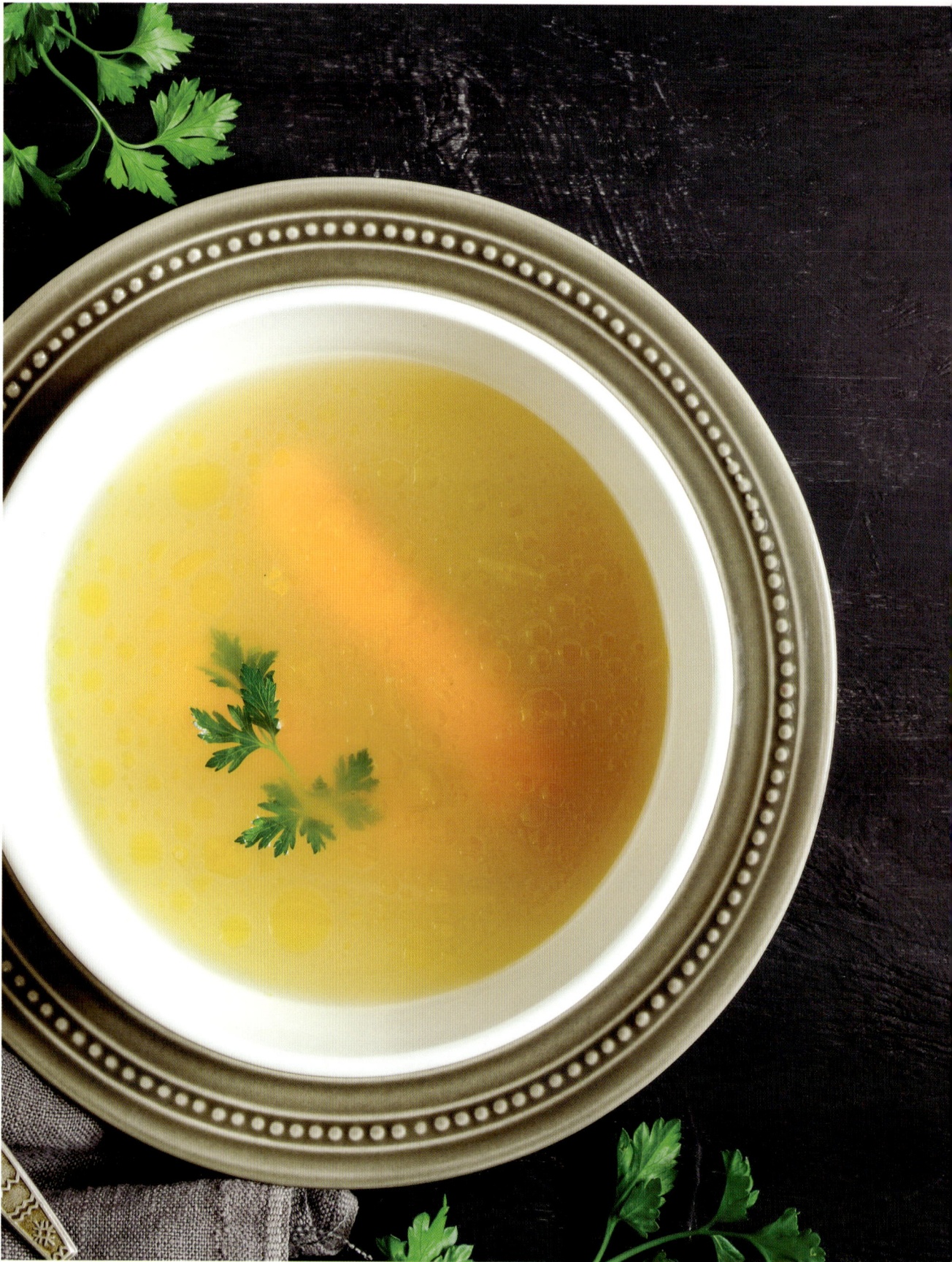

CHICKEN STOCK

Makes 2–3 litres (70–102 fl oz)

- × 2 tablespoons vegetable oil
- × 2 kg (4 lb 8 oz) chicken carcass (wings, skin, bones, etc.)
- × 2 onions, halved
- × 3 carrots, halved
- × 5 garlic cloves, unpeeled
- × 2 bay leaves
- × 10 black peppercorns
- × 2 celery stalks, leaves included, roughly chopped
- × sea salt

METHOD

Preheat the oven to 180°C (350°F/Gas 4). Grease a baking tray with 1 tablespoon of the vegetable oil. Put the chicken on the tray. Add the onion, carrot and garlic cloves. Drizzle the remaining vegetable oil over the top and roast until lightly browned and spluttering with roasted goodness.

Place the roasted chicken and vegetables into a stockpot over low heat (use a little water to scrape all of the brown and burnt bits from the pan and add to the pot as well). Add 6 litres (203 fl oz) of water to the pot. Add the bay leaves, peppercorns and celery.

Simmer for 3 hours, skimming the scum off the top every 30 minutes. Remove from the heat and allow to cool slightly.

Pass the stock through a fine mesh sieve into a large glass bowl or metal pot. Season with sea salt.

Place in the fridge for 1 hour and remove the layer of fat from the surface. Store in batches in the freezer for 4-6 months.

BEEF STOCK

Makes 2–3 litres (70–102 fl oz)

- × 2 tablespoons olive oil
- × 2 kg (4 lb 8 oz) beef bones
- × 2 onions, halved
- × 3 carrots, halved
- × 5 garlic cloves, unpeeled
- × 2 bay leaves

- × 10 black peppercorns
- × 2 celery stalks, leaves included, roughly chopped
- × 3 thyme sprigs
- × 3 flat-leaf (Italian) parsley sprigs
- × sea salt

METHOD

Preheat the oven to 180°C (350°F/Gas 4). Grease a baking tray with 1 tablespoon of the vegetable oil. Put the beef on the tray. Add the onion, carrot and garlic cloves. Drizzle the remaining vegetable oil over the top and roast until lightly browned and spluttering with roasted goodness.

Place the roasted beef bones and vegetables into a stockpot over low heat (use a little water to scrape all of the brown and burnt bits from the pan and add to the pot as well). Add 6 litres (203 fl oz) of water to the pot. Add the bay leaves, peppercorns, thyme, flat-leaf parsley and celery.

Simmer for 3 hours, skimming the scum off the top every 30 minutes. Remove from the heat and allow to cool slightly.

Pass the stock through a fine mesh sieve into a large glass bowl or metal pot. Season with sea salt.

Place in the fridge for 1 hour and remove the layer of fat from the surface. Store in batches in the freezer for 4-6 months.

FISH STOCK

Makes 2–3 litres (70–102 fl oz)

- × 2 tablespoons vegetable oil
- × 2 kg (4 lb 8 oz) fish carcass (you can buy these from your local fishmonger. Prawn heads and shells are good for this as well)
- × 2 onions, halved
- × 3 carrots, halved
- × 5 garlic cloves, unpeeled
- × 2 lime leaves
- × 30 g (1 oz) ginger
- × 5 coriander (cilantro) sprigs
- × 10 black peppercorns
- × 2 celery stalks, leaves included, chopped
- × sea salt

METHOD

Preheat the oven to 180 °C (350 °F/Gas 4). Grease a baking tray with 1 tablespoon of the vegetable oil. Put the fish pieces on the tray. Add the onion, carrot and garlic cloves. Drizzle the remaining vegetable oil over the top and roast until lightly browned and spluttering with roasted goodness.

Place the fish and vegetables into a stockpot over low heat (use a little water to scrape all of the brown and burnt bits from the pan and add to the pot as well). Add 6 litres (203 fl oz) of water to the pot. Add the ginger, lime leaves, coriander, peppercorns and celery.

Simmer for 3 hours, skimming the scum off the top every 30 minutes. Remove from the heat and allow to cool slightly.

Pass the stock through a fine mesh sieve into a large glass bowl or metal pot. Season with sea salt.

Place in the fridge for 1 hour and remove the layer of fat from the surface. Store in batches in the freezer for 4-6 months.

CHILLI SAMBAL

Makes 150 g (51/2 oz)

- × 100 g (3½ oz) long red chillies, roughly chopped
- × 30 g (1 oz) ginger, peeled and grated
- × 6 garlic cloves, finely sliced
- × 1 tablespoon dried chilli flakes
- × 1 tablespoon sugar
- × 1 teaspoon salt
- × 2 tablespoons fish sauce
- × 125 ml (4 fl oz) vegetable oil

METHOD

Place the chillies, ginger, garlic, chilli flakes, sugar, salt, fish sauce and vegetable oil into a food processor and blend well, stopping to scrape down the sides with a plastic spatula, ensuring there are no large chunks.

Transfer the chilli mixture to a saucepan and heat over medium heat until mixture starts to bubble. Reduce the heat to low and cook for 20 minzutes, stirring to ensure mixture does not stick or burn. (This can smell a little like someone has let off pepper spray in the house so make sure your windows are open and pets and small children are out of the room!)

Remove from the heat and allow to cool. Transfer the chilli sambal an airtight container in the refrigerator for 5 days (or portion the mixture and you can freeze it for up to 3-4 months).

RED CURRY PASTE

Makes 125 g (4½ oz)

INGREDIENTS

- × 7 dried red long chillies, stems removed, deseeded and roughly chopped
- × 1 teaspoon ground coriander seed
- × 1 teaspoon ground cumin
- × 7 long red chillies, stems removed, deseeded and roughly chopped
- × 25 g (1 oz) galangal, finely diced
- × 2 lemongrass stalks, thinly sliced
- × 6 garlic cloves, crushed
- × 5 kaffir lime leaves, finely chopped
- × 4 shallots, finely chopped
- × 4 coriander (cilantro) roots, finely chopped
- × ¼ bunch coriander (cilantro), finely chopped
- × 2 teaspoons shrimp paste
- × 1 tablespoon fish sauce
- × 1 teaspoon brown sugar
- × 1 teaspoon black pepper
- × 1 teaspoon sea salt

METHOD

Pour 125 ml (4 fl oz) hot water into a bowl and immerse the dried chillies, soaking until soft (about 10 minutes). Set aside on a paper towel to drain.

Heat the coriander seed and cumin in a small frypan over low heat until fragrant. Transfer to a mixing bowl. Add the remaining ingredients.

Now, you have two choices here: you can either use a mortar and pestle to pound and grind the ingredients into a paste, or use a blender or food processor. Whichever method you choose, make sure you don't leave any chunks in the paste.

Store in an airtight container in the refrigerator for 3-5 days (or portion the mixture and you can freeze it for up to 3-4 months).

HUMMUS

Makes 300 g (10½ oz)

- × 400 g (14 oz) tinned chickpeas
- × juice of 1 lemon
- × 3 garlic cloves, roughly chopped
- × 1½ tablespoons sesame oil
- × 4 tablespoons olive oil
- × 2 teaspoons smoked paprika
- × sea salt and cracked black pepper, to season

METHOD

Place all the ingredients into a food processor. Blend until smooth.

Store in an airtight container in the refrigerator for 3 days (or you can freeze the mixture for up to 3-4 months).

TZATZIKI

Makes 300 g (10½ oz)

- × ½ Lebanese (short) cucumber, cut into quarters lengthways
- × 2 garlic cloves, crushed
- × 1½ tablespoons chopped dill
- × juice of ½ lemon
- × 225 g (8 oz) Greek yoghurt
- × 3 tablespoons olive oil
- × ½ teaspoon sea salt

METHOD

Lay each cucumber quarter on a chopping board and run your knife carefully down the flesh of the cucumber, just behind the seeds. Discard the seeds and repeat with the remaining cucumber. Chop the cucumber into small pieces and place into a mixing bowl.

Add the remaining ingredients to the bowl and gently mix to combine.

Store in an airtight container in the refrigerator for 2 days.

MOTHER'S DAY

There's a strange scene that plays out against the cold, dark streets as the first strains of dawn break across the sky on Mother's Day each year, and it was only recently that I was privy to this extraordinary annual oddity.

Like most women, when asked what she wanted for Mother's Day my wife replied with the almost universal response, 'a sleep-in please'. I, of course, heartily agreed and promised a breakfast to remember, assuring her I would take care of everything.

And up until I lay down in bed the night before, I thought I had.

While I had managed to secure a gift on behalf of my daughter (my wrapping skills so poor it actually looked like an infant had done it) I, like the moron that I am, failed to remember to get the ingredients for the promised breakfast in bed. So I fashioned a brilliant plan to get up and out of the house as soon as my little girl stirred to secure the ingredients for this feast, while my wife remained blissfully asleep and none the wiser.

At first light, I hastily dressed and packed my little one into her pram, leaving the house in search of an open store or supermarket. As we made our way down the darkened streets I noticed a curious and unexpected sight.

The streets which I thought would be all but deserted were in fact populated by men.

This was a strange sight to behold and the absence of the fairer sex was noticeable. It was as if I was in the fictional town of Hamelin and the Pied Piper had spirited away the women instead of the town's children.

When I arrived at the brightly lit supermarket at the end of my street I was greeted with a similar scene, herds of bleary eyed and confused of fathers desperately combing the aisles in search of ingredients, their children in various states of dress and grooming, bewildered and complaining as to why they had been dragged out of the house so early.

And while I found this unusual and unspoken phenomenon (known only to fathers, half asleep children and shopkeepers) most amusing, I could not help but feel for those few poor souls who had woken in the middle of the night sitting bolt upright in bed, realising they had forgotten Mother's Day all together. You could tell who they were straight away, they had an air of desperation about them as they raced wild eyed from aisle to aisle with a basket filled with random items, hoping to hell that nothing says 'I Love You' more than a block of chocolate and a can of air freshener—the best they could find on offer at 6am.

Luckily for those of us with less than perfect memories, most supermarkets now actually plan for our stupidity and stock fresh flowers and cards, which are available for purchase before the sun has even risen.

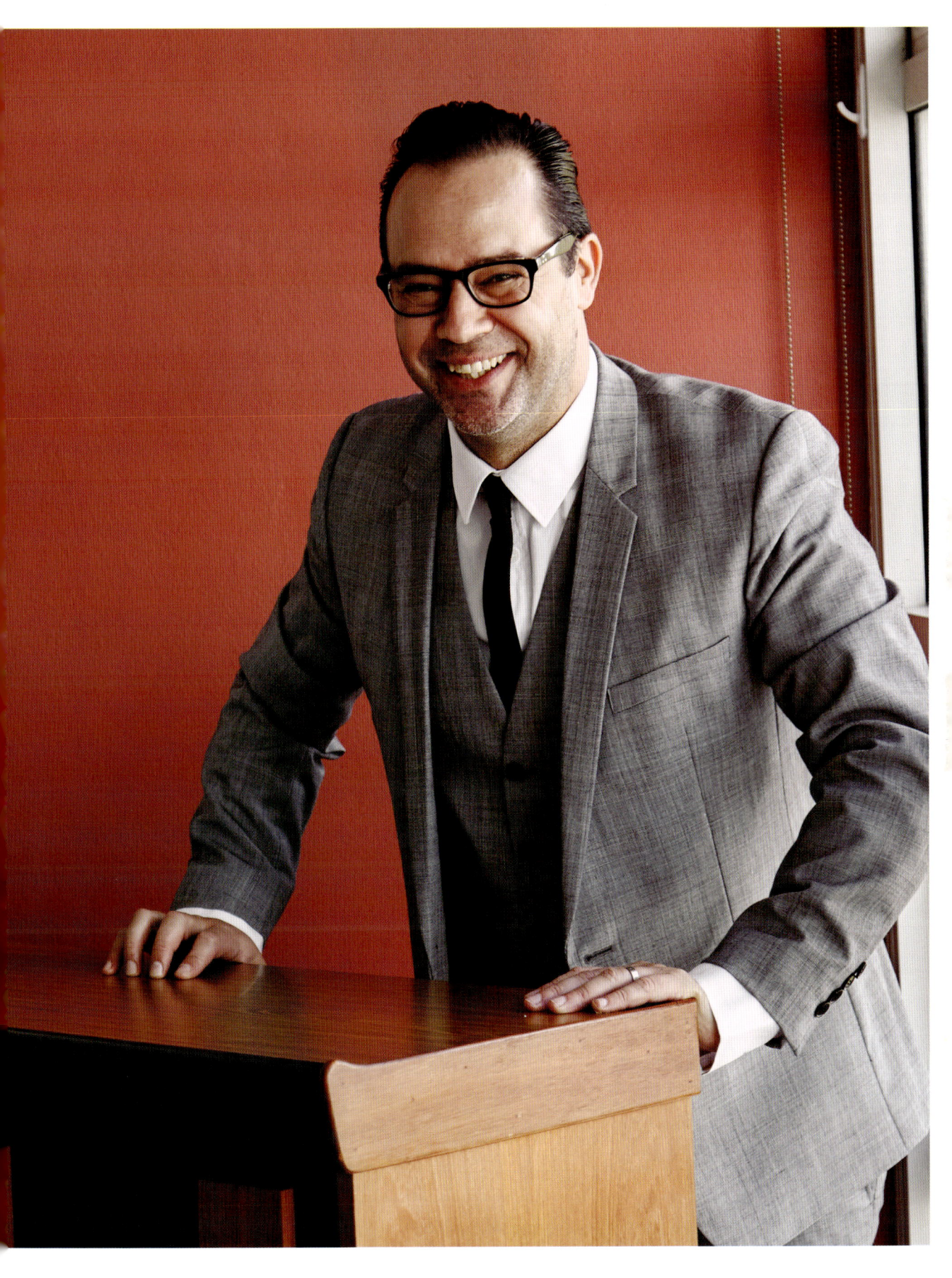

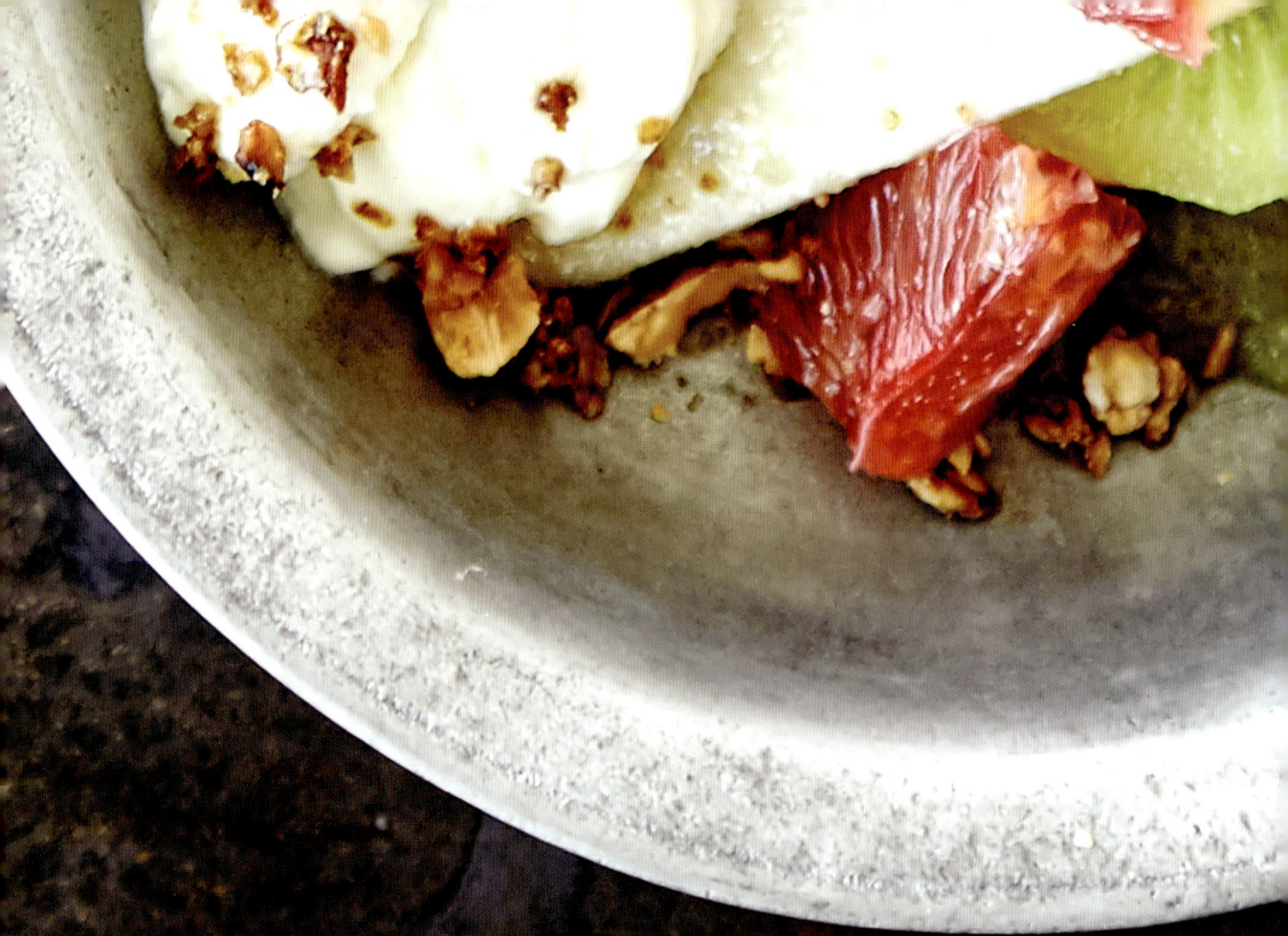

FIRST THING IN THE MORNING

A few worthwhile ideas for dragging yourself out of bed early

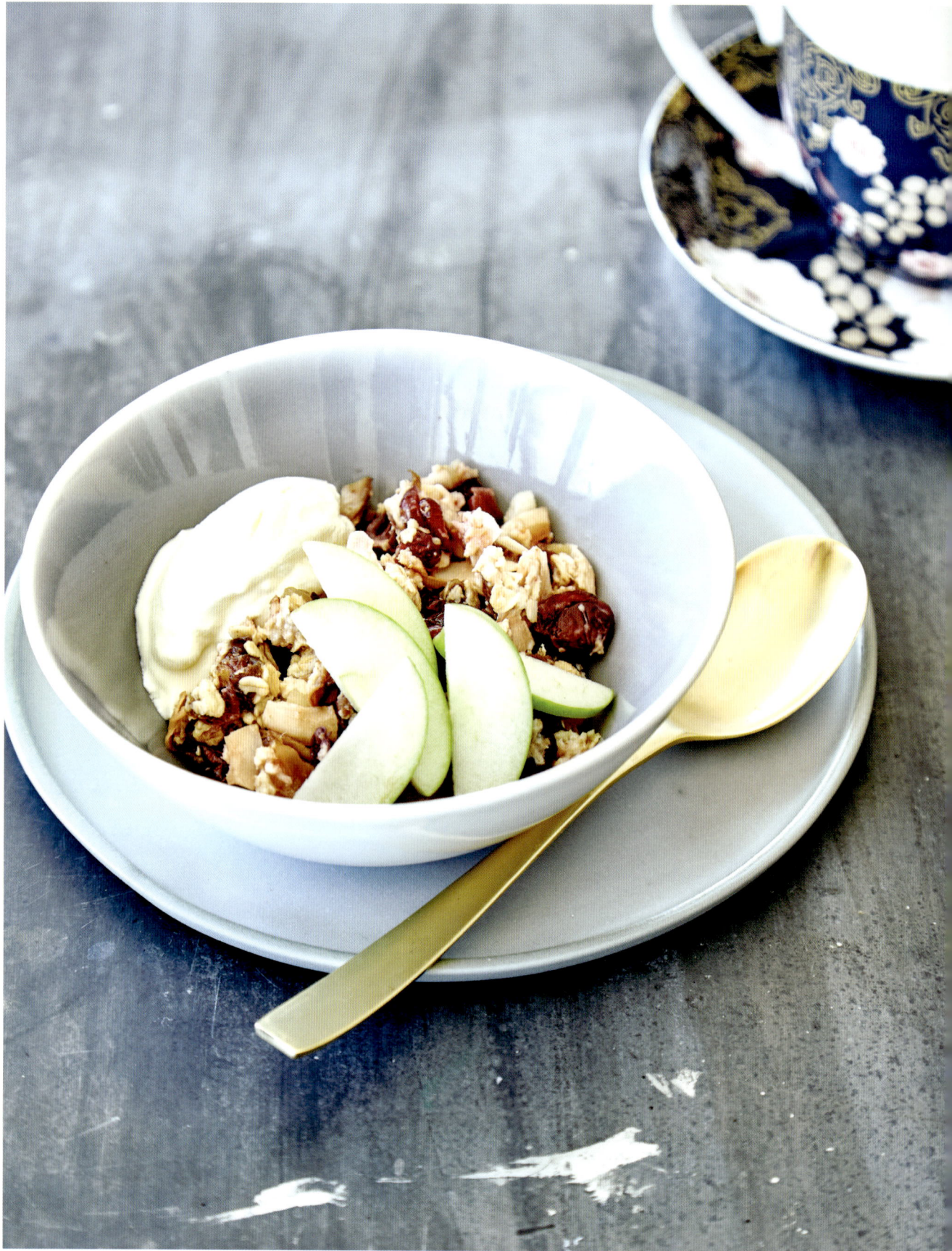

Muesli is a delicious way to start the day and the great thing is it's got most of the things a pregnant woman needs for a healthy breakfast, like nuts, fruit and diary. The problem with a lot of store-bought muesli is that on closer examination most products are high in fat and sugar. The best thing about homemade muesli is you can choose what goes in. I have used apples, figs and cranberry but if you don't like any of the fruit and nuts you can simply mix and match—after all, you're the one making it!

FIG, CRANBERRY & MACADAMIA MUESLI

Serves 2
Cooking Time: Overnight + 10 minutes

INGREDIENTS

- × 25 g (1 oz) macadamia nuts
- × 2 tablespoons shredded coconut
- × 30 g (1 oz) dried figs, chopped
- × 100 g (3½ oz) rolled (porridge) oats
- × 30 g (1 oz) dried cranberries
- × 125 ml (4 fl oz) apple juice
- × 1 apple
- × ¼ teaspoon cinnamon
- × 125 ml (4 fl oz) natural yogurt
- × 1 tablespoon maple syrup

METHOD

Using a rolling pin, place the macadamia nuts under a clean tea towel and roughly crush them.

Heat a small frying pan over medium heat and toast the macadamia nuts and coconut until fragrant. Remove from the heat and add to a mixing bowl.

Add the figs, rolled oats, dried cranberries and apple juice. Place the bowl in the fridge overnight.

When ready to serve, cut the apple into bite-sized pieces and sprinkle with the cinnamon.

Remove the oat mixture from the fridge divide into two bowls, adding half the yoghurt to each bowl. Top with the apple and drizzle with the maple syrup.

Omelettes are a great way to serve eggs well-done for your pregnant partner and you can pack them full of great ingredients so they get a healthy start to the day. Varieties of the humble omelette are as varied as your imagination, I have chosen pan-fried mushrooms with baby English spinach and thyme but it can also be something as simple like a classic French omelette with fresh chervil, parsley and grated gruyère to something totally indulgent like the American classic Denver omelette with ham, bacon, cheese and green capsicum. Whichever type of omelette you make, just be sure to cook the egg through. For a great breakfast serve with a Fruit salad (see page 63) and a Shake (see page 67-68).

PAN FRIED MUSHROOM OMELETTE WITH SPINACH AND THYME

Serves 2
Cooking Time: 20 minutes

INGREDIENTS

- × olive oil, for cooking
- × 200 g (7 oz) mushrooms (any type you like), thinly sliced
- × 50 g (13/4 oz) baby English spinach, roughly chopped
- × 1 thyme sprig, leaves picked and chopped
- × 3 eggs
- × 1 tablespoon unsalted butter
- × 30 g (1 oz) cheddar cheese
- × sea salt and cracked black pepper, to season

METHOD

Heat a drizzle of olive oil in a non-stick frying pan over medium heat. Add the mushrooms and cook until browned. Add the baby English spinach and thyme and cook until the spinach is wilted. Remove the pan from the heat, season well with salt and pepper and set aside.

Place the eggs into a bowl and whisk. Heat the butter in a non-stick frying pan over medium heat, allowing it to melt and foam. Pour the eggs into the pan and let them cook until the bottom has started to brown and the egg is only slightly liquid on the top.

Add the mushrooms and spinach to one side of the egg mixture and grate the cheese over the top.

Using a spatula, fold one side of the omelette over, covering the mushrooms and spinach. Cook until the eggs are fully cooked through. Remove from the heat, cut in half and serve immediately.

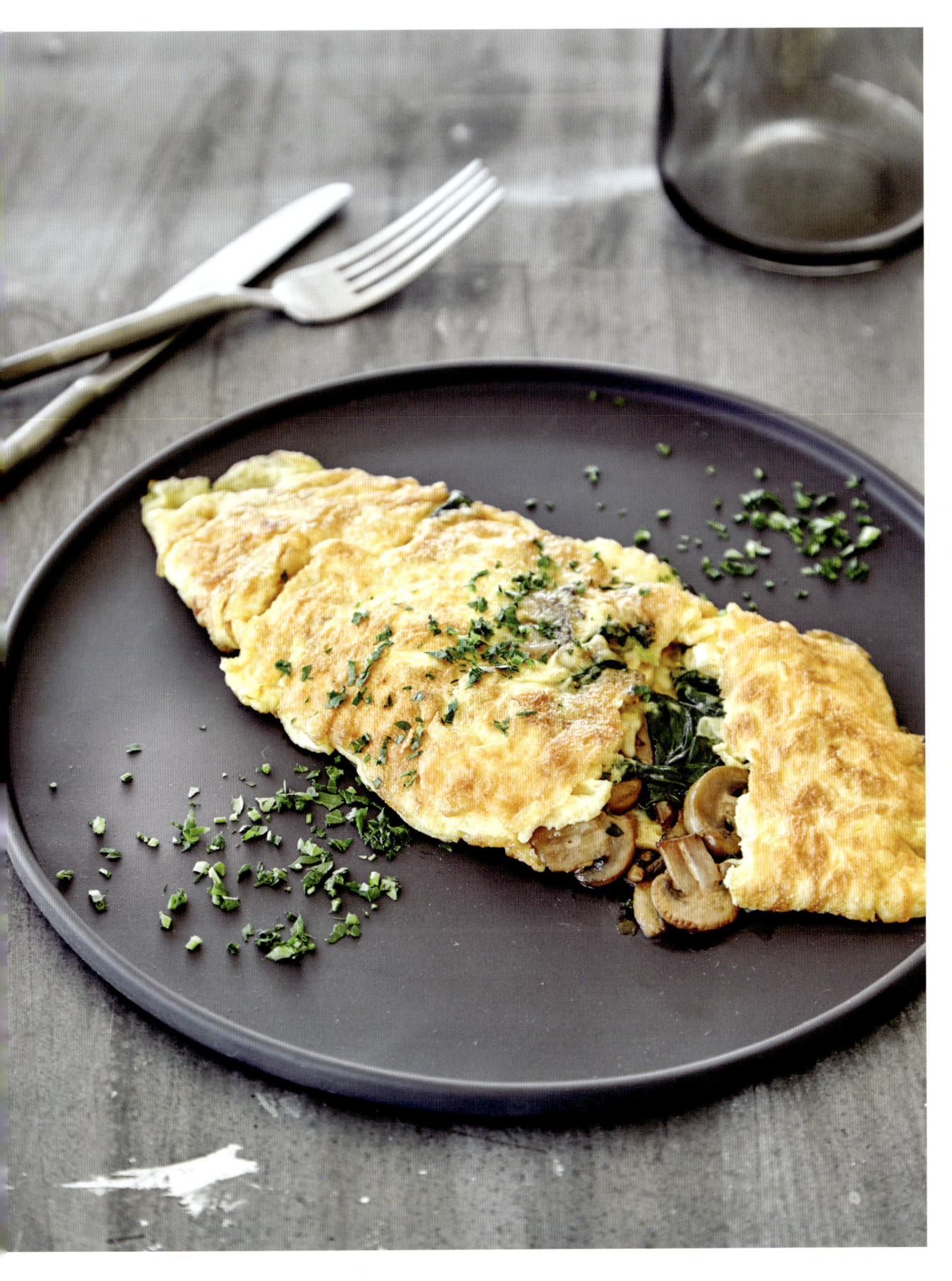

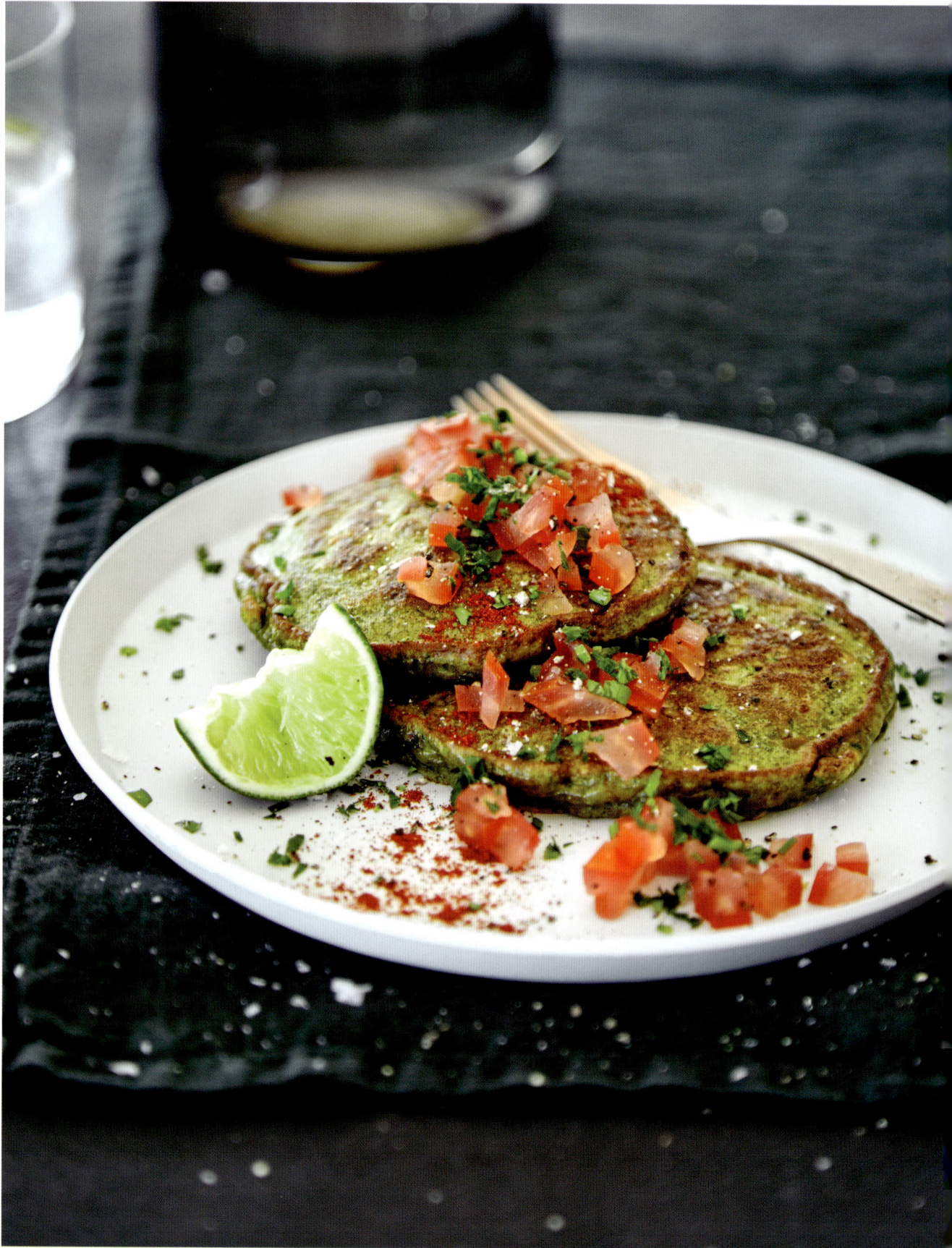

Sometimes you feel like something different than the run-of-the-mill fruit or cereal or eggs or toast for breakfast and who can blame you? Having the same things day in and day out is bound to send even the most balanced and even tempered among us round the bend. Well if you're looking for something different for breakfast look no further than these corn fritters and with the spinach blended into the batter so you won't even know it's good for you!

CORN & RED ONION FRITTERS

Serves 4
Cooking Time: 20 minutes

INGREDIENTS

- × 3 corn cobs
- × olive oil, for cooking
- × 1 red onion, cut into thin slices
- × 1 tablespoon maple syrup, plus extra for drizzling
- × 50 g (13/4 oz) baby English spinach
- × 3 tablespoons milk

- × 2 eggs
- × 125 g (4½ oz) plain (all-purpose) flour
- × 1 teaspoon baking powder
- × 1 teaspoon bicarbonate of soda (baking soda)
- × 2 teaspoons chipotle powder or smoked paprika
- × sea salt and cracked black pepper, to season

METHOD

Hold each cob vertically on the chopping board, running a knife down each side and slicing off all of the kernels. Repeat on each cob of corn.

Heat the olive oil in a frying pan over low heat. Add the corn and onion and cook until the onions are soft. Increase the heat to high and cook until the corn and onion starts to colour and blacken. Pour in the maple syrup and cook until the sugar caramelizes. Remove from the heat and set aside.

Place the spinach, milk and eggs into a food processor and blend until combined. Add the flour, baking powder, bicarbonate of soda and chipotle powder or smoked paprika to the blender and combine. Pour the mixture into a bowl and add the corn and the onions. Season well with salt and pepper.

Heat the olive oil in a frying pan over medium heat. When hot, add several tablespoons of the fritter batter to the pan ensuring they are well spaced.

Cook until golden, then turn over the fritters and continue cooking until golden. Remove the fritters from the pan and drain on a paper towel, repeating the steps with the rest of the batter.

Serve the corn fritters warm, with maple syrup, if you like.

There is nothing better than homemade baked beans. I don't know why they are so good but they just are and once you get a taste for them you'll wonder why you ever bothered with the tinned version at all. I have added kale to this recipe so we can put some extra folates and iron into the dish but as always feel free to experiment and come up with your own combinations.

SCRAMBLED EGGS WITH HOMEMADE BAKED BEANS

Serves 4
Cooking Time: 30 minutes

INGREDIENTS

BAKED BEANS & KALE

× 400 g (14 oz) tinned crushed tomatoes
× olive oil, for cooking
× 1 teaspoon tomato paste (concentrated purée)
× 1½ teaspoons smoked paprika
× 2 teaspoons soft brown sugar
× 400 g (14 oz) tinned cannellini beans, drained
× 50 g (13/4 oz) kale
× sea salt and cracked black pepper, to season

× SCRAMBLED EGGS

× 6 eggs
× 3 tablespoons low-fat milk
× 1 tablespoon unsalted butter

× 4 slices of bread (see note)
× 12 cherry tomatoes, roughly chopped
× sea salt and cracked black pepper, to season

METHOD

Place the crushed tomatoes in a mixing bowl and break up any large chunks using a potato masher.

Heat the olive oil in a saucepan over medium heat. When hot, add the tomato paste, smoked paprika and sugar and stir until fragrant. Add the beans and tomatoes and mix to combine. Season with sea salt and cracked black pepper.

Bring to the boil and then reduce the heat to a simmer and cook for 15 minutes, stirring to ensure nothing sticks to the bottom. Season if necessary, then add the kale and cook for a further 5 minutes. Remove from the heat and set aside.

Break the eggs into a mixing bowl and add the milk, whisking together well.

Heat the butter in a non-stick frying pan over medium heat until it melts and begins to foam. Add the egg mixture and let it sit in the pan for about ten seconds before pushing the mixture to towards the centre from the outside, using a wooden spoon. Continue doing this until the eggs are fully cooked and fluffy. (Normally scrambled eggs are taken off while still sightly runny and underdone but for safety reasons it is important to ensure they are cooked fully thorough). Set aside.

Toast the bread, then place on a plate and top with baked beans and eggs. Garnish with the chopped cherry tomatoes and season with sea salt and cracked black pepper. Serve immediately.

Note: If you are using packaged bread, check the ingredients as they normally add folic acid and iodine which are two essentials.

Funtastic Baby Facts
Did you know a baby has 6-8 wet diapers every day?

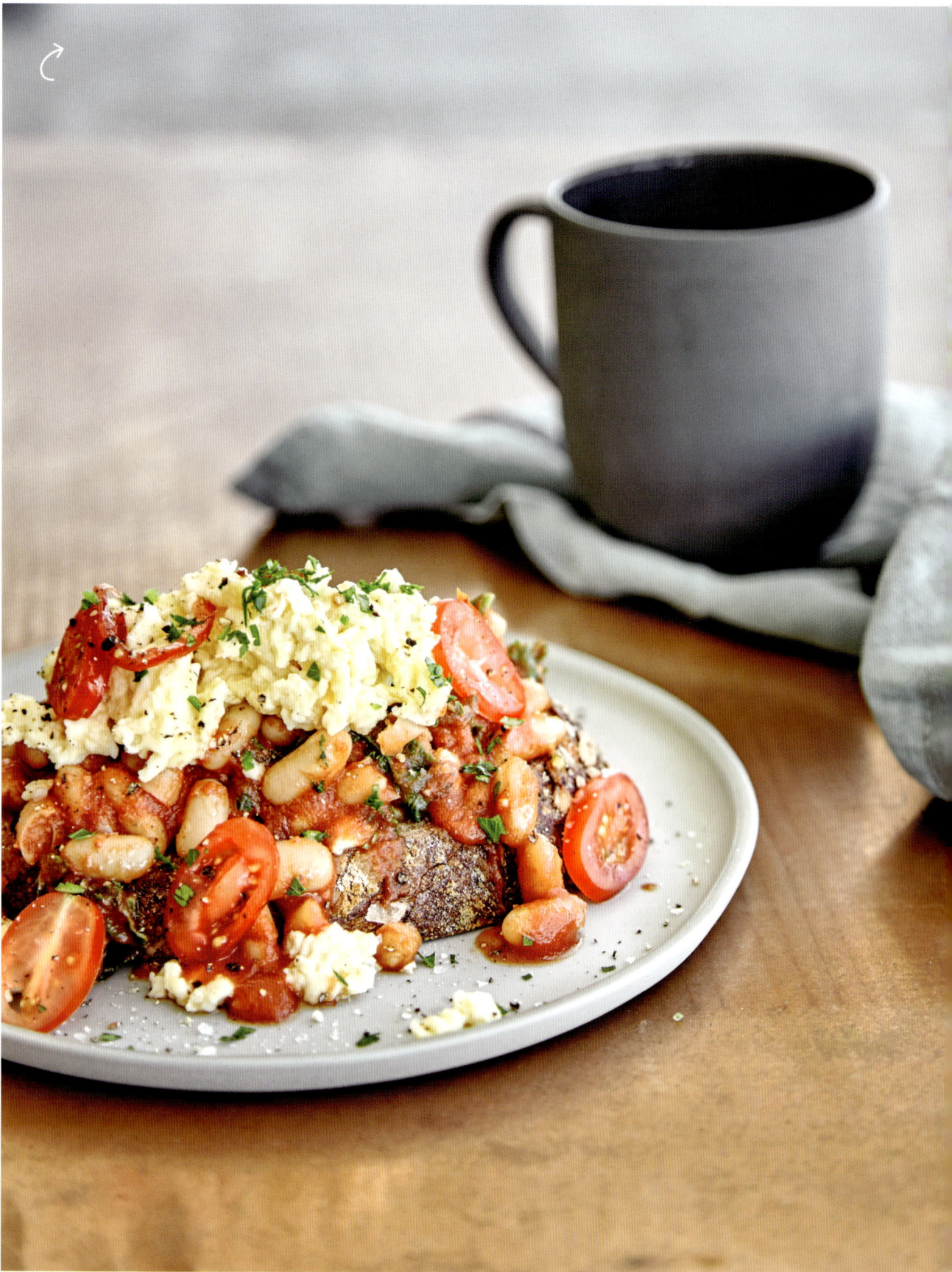

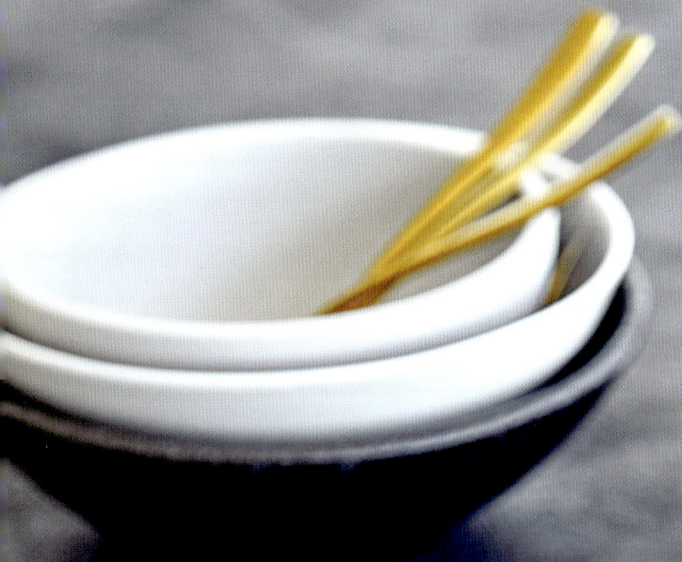

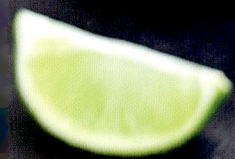

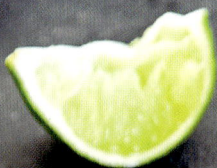

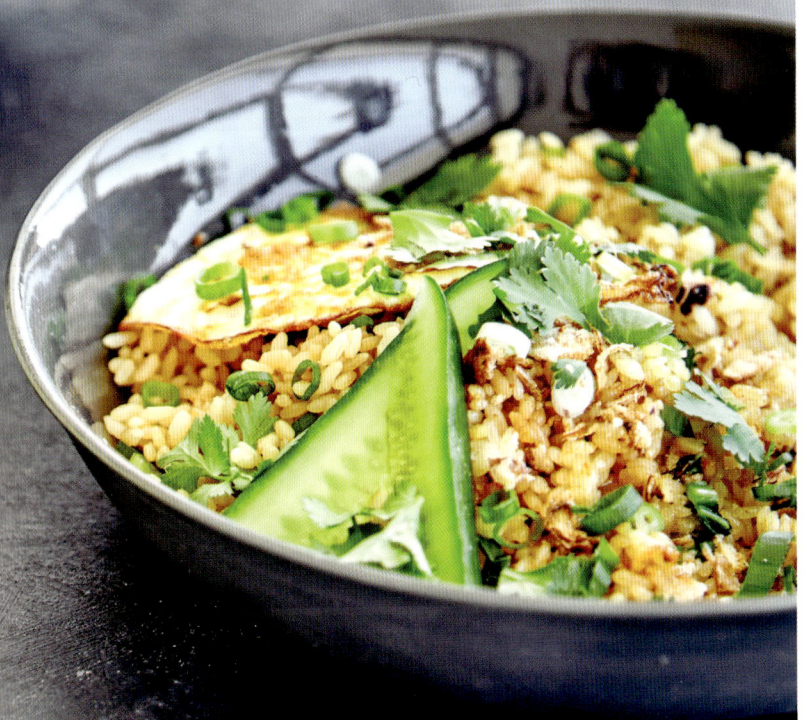

This is one of those dishes that requires a little forethought so for best results you need to make the rice the night before and store in the fridge. Traditional Nasi goreng does not normally have the meat and seafood that you might find in this dish when eating at a restaurant but instead is served quite simply. Feel free to mix up the ingredients if you want more greens and if you need to tone it down, omit the chillies and sambal.

NASI GORENG

Serves 4
Cooking Time: Overnight plus 25 minutes

INGREDIENTS

RICE
- × 125 g (41/2 oz) rice
- × 125 ml (4 fl oz) chicken stock (see Basics, page 31 or use unsalted if store-bought)
- × 3 tablespoons light soy sauce
- × 25 g (1 oz) ginger, finely chopped
- × 2 garlic cloves, crushed
- × 1 red chilli, finely sliced
- × ½ teaspoons shrimp paste
- × ½ teaspoons palm sugar
- × vegetable oil, for cooking

- × 4 eggs
- × 2 tablespoons chilli sambal (optional, see Basics, page 34)
- × 1 bunch choy sum, finely chopped
- × 1 spring onion (scallion) stalk, finely chopped
- × 1 tablespoon kecap manis
- × 4 tablespoons fried shallots
- × ¼ bunch coriander (cilantro), roughly chopped
- × 2 Lebanese (short) cucumbers, sliced lengthways, to garnish

Place the rice in a rice cooker and cover with chicken stock and light soy sauce. Cook as per instructions until done. Alternatively, place the rice in a saucepan, add the light soy sauce and cover with double the amount of chicken stock listed, then bring to boil. Reduce the heat to a simmer and cook until the stock is absorbed and rice is tender yet firm (about 10-15 minutes).

Leave for 10 minutes, then remove the rice and spread over a baking tray. Place in the fridge to cool overnight. The next day, remove the rice from the fridge and break up any clumps.

Place the ginger, garlic, chilli, shrimp paste and palm sugar into a mortar and pound into a paste with a pestle (If you don't own one just mix together well in a bowl).

Heat the vegetable oil in a frying pan over medium heat. When hot, crack in the eggs.

When fried, flip over carefully and fry the other side, ensuring the yolks are cooked through and the egg is well done. Transfer the eggs to a plate and cover with foil.

Heat the vegetable oil in a wok over medium heat. When hot, add the ginger, garlic and chilli mixture and cook until fragrant. Add the chilli sambal (if using) and stir for a further 30 seconds. Add the choy sum and cook until wilted.

Add the rice, spring onion and kecap manis and continue to move the rice in the wok until the choy sum is well distributed and the kecap manis and the ginger, garlic and chilli mixture coats the rice.

Divide the rice between four bowls, top with a fried egg, a crumble of fried shallots and garnish with coriander and cucumber slices.

One of the best ways to add flavour to things is to roast them. Science calls it the Maillard reaction but to you and me It's the brown, crunchy goodness that unlocks hundreds of hidden dark and delicious flavors. You will see throughout this book that I roast a lot of the ingredients for that exact reason, but if it is too time consuming and you want to skip that part of the recipe pleased go right ahead (that is unless you are cooking the roast chicken later on in the book, then I'd stick to the recipe). For these muffins we are combining the sweet flavours of roasted pumpkin, carrot and apples with the earthiness of wholemeal flour, cinnamon and olive oil.

ROASTED PUMPKIN, CARROT & APPLE MUFFINS WITH OLIVE OIL AND CUMIN

Makes 12
Cooking Time: 1 hour

INGREDIENTS

- × 2 tablespoons balsamic vinegar
- × 2 tablespoons honey
- × 500 g (1 lb 2 oz) pumpkin flesh, roughly chopped
- × 500 g (1 lb 2 oz) carrots, roughly chopped
- × 500 g (1 lb 2 oz) apples, peeled and roughly chopped
- × 125 g (4½ oz) plain (all-purpose) flour
- × 2 teaspoons baking powder
- × 1 teaspoon bicarbonate of soda (baking soda)

- × 125 g (4½ oz) wholemeal (whole-wheat) flour
- × 30g (1 oz) wheat germ
- × ½ teaspoons salt
- × 1 teaspoon cumin
- × 1½ teaspoons ground cinnamon
- × 75 g (3 oz) soft brown sugar
- × 2 eggs
- × 3 tablespoons olive oil

(continued

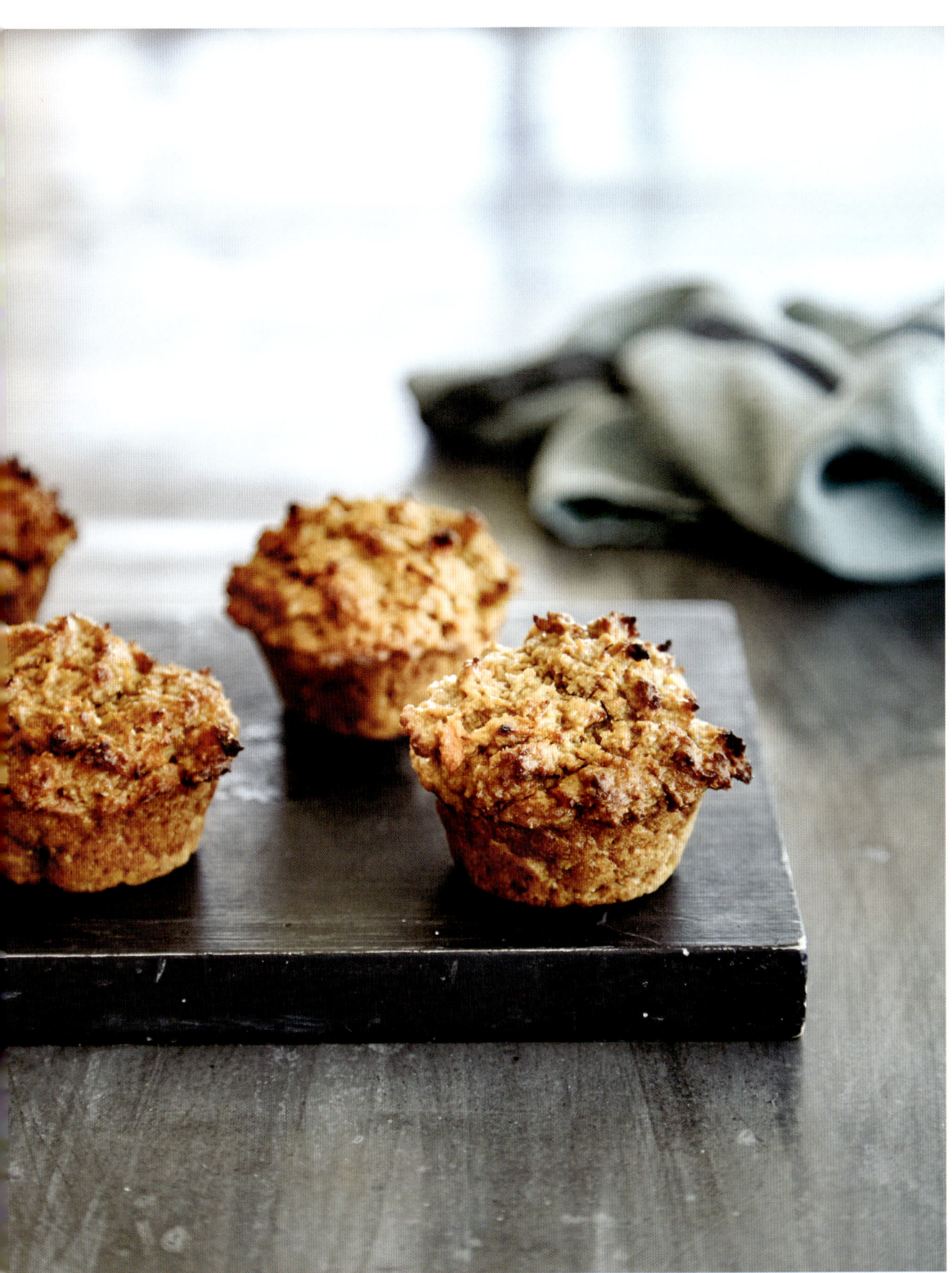

ROASTED PUMPKIN, CARROT & APPLE MUFFINS WITH OLIVE OIL AND CUMIN CONTINUED...

Preheat the oven to 190°C (375°F). Lightly grease a 12-hole muffin tin and baking tray.

Combine the balsamic vinegar and honey in a bowl and set aside.

Toss the pumpkin, carrot and apples pieces in the balsamic vinegar and honey mixture and lay them on the baking tray. Roast in the oven until browned. Remove from the oven and leave to cool slightly.

Place the roast pumpkin, carrot and apples in a food processor and purée until smooth (you may need to do this in batches.

Place the purée into a large mixing bowl and set aside until needed.

Sift the plain flour, baking powder and bicarbonate of soda into a large bowl. Add the wholemeal flour, wheat germ, salt, cumin, cinnamon and brown sugar and mix together well.

Add the eggs into a separate large bowl and whisk.

Add the purée and the olive oil to the egg mixture and stir until combined.

Pour the flour mixture into the wet ingredients and fold together with a rubber spatula (do not overmix the batter).

Pour the batter into the muffin holes (they should be about two-thirds full) and bake for about 18 minutes. Check to see if they are cooked by inserting a bamboo skewer into the top, if there's no raw batter, they are done.

Leave to cool for about 5 minutes. Serve with butter, or for an awesome savoury treat, a spread of Hummus (see Basics, page 36).

Store in an airtight container in the refrigerator 3-4 days (or you can freeze the mixture for up to 6-8 months).

Another easy way to pack a sweet with flavour is the addition of herbs and spices, we do it all the time with savoury but for some reason seem to forget about it when it comes to the sweet stuff. I have used cardamom and cinnamon to spice up the apples and strawberries but feel free to experiment and come up with your own combinations. Just remember, if you are adding spices to a meal make sure you take the time a dry-roast them in a frying pan—it only takes a minute or so to do but it brings the ingredient to life (some spices sit on shelves for quite some time before ever finding their way into your pantry). If you take the time and do this simple little step, you will infuse your dishes with flavour every time.

BUCKWHEAT MUFFINS WITH STRAWBERRY, APPLE AND YOGHURT

Makes 12
Cooking Time: 40 minutes

INGREDIENTS

- × 50 g (13/4 oz) pistachios
- × 2 teaspoons ground cardamom
- × 2 teaspoons ground cinnamon
- × 125 g (4½ oz) apples, peeled and finely diced
- × 190 g (63/4 oz) strawberries, hulled and roughly chopped
- × 40 g (11/2 oz) soft brown sugar
- × 65 g (21/4 oz) plain (all-purpose) flour

- × 1 teaspoon baking powder
- × ½ teaspoons bicarbonate of soda (baking soda)
- × 100 g (3½ oz) buckwheat flour
- × ½ teaspoon salt
- × 1 egg
- × 190 ml (6½ fl oz) plain yoghurt
- × 30 ml (1 fl oz) olive oil

Continued ⟶

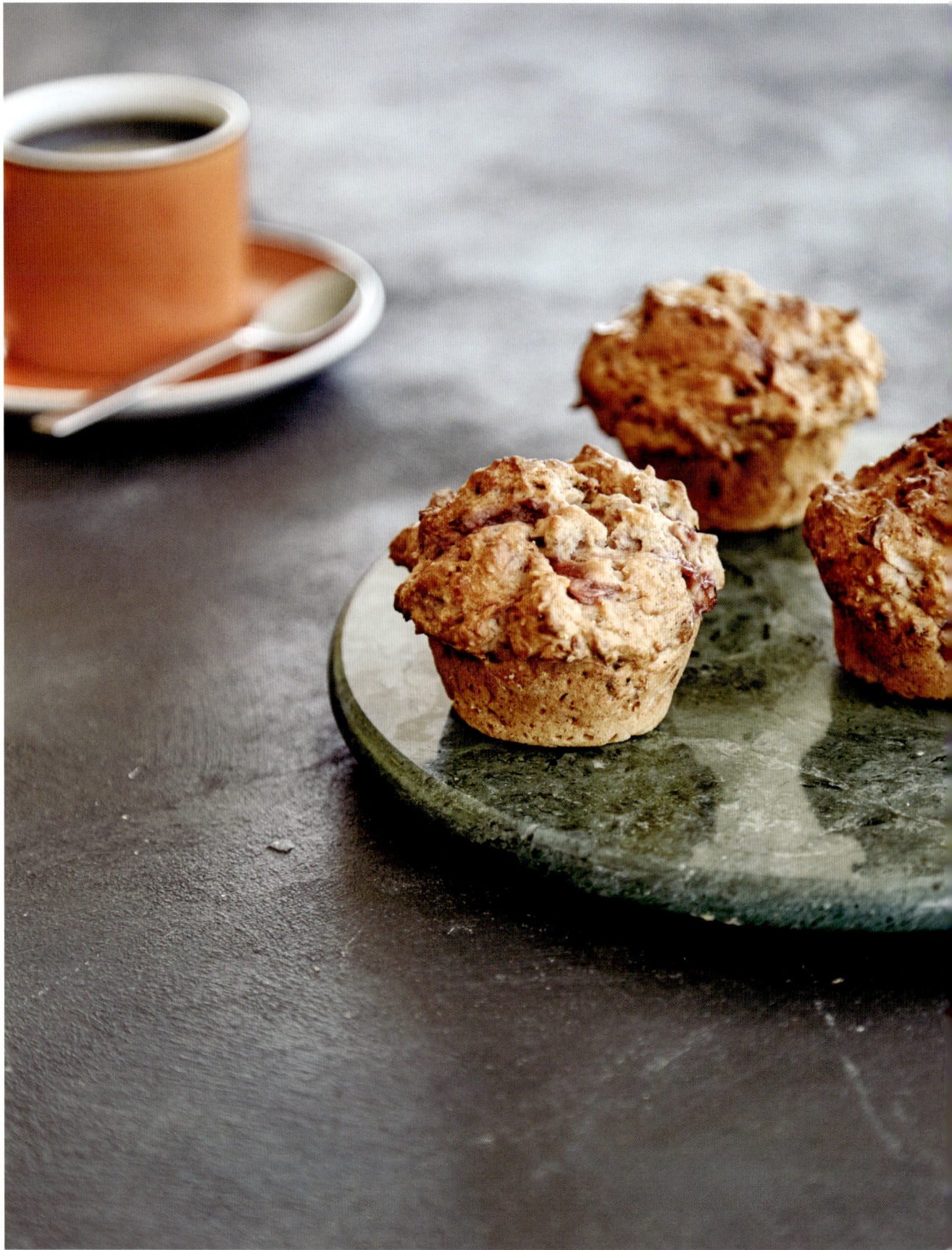

BUCKWHEAT MUFFINS WITH STRAWBERRY, APPLE AND YOGHURT CONTINUED...

Preheat the oven to 180°C (375°F). Lightly grease a 12-hole muffin tin.

Roughly crush the pistachios with a rolling pin. Place a dry frying pan over low heat and add the pistachios, cardamom and cinnamon. Cook until fragrant then remove to a small mixing bowl.

Toss the apples in the pistachio mix, coating well. Set aside until needed.

Place the strawberries, sugar and 2 tablespoons of water in a saucepan over low heat. Cook for 15 minutes, or until the strawberries are soft and break down. Remove from the heat and allow to cool.

Add the plain flour, baking powder, bicarbonate of soda, buckwheat flour and salt to a large mixing bowl and combine well.

In a separate bowl, add the egg and whisk. Add the strawberry coulis, yoghurt, apple pieces, pistachios, olive oil and mix together until combined.

Pour the flour mixture into the wet ingredients and fold together with a rubber spatula (do not overmix the batter).

Pour the batter into the muffin holes (they should be about three-quarters full) and bake for 15 minutes. Check to see if they are cooked by inserting a bamboo skewer into the top, if there's no raw batter, they are done. Leave to cool for about 5 minutes, then serve.

Note: Store in an airtight container in the refrigerator 3-4 days (or you can freeze the mixture for up to 6-8 months).

So, in the little time you have left before this tradition goes by the wayside I would suggest you give your partner a bit of a treat and wake up early to make them breakfast in bed. You can go for the more traditional Sunday breakfast of bacon and eggs or, if you want to mix it up, I would suggest dropping this breakfast staple off the menu all together and replacing it with one of my personal favourites, pancakes!

You can make your pancakes from many different ingredients and the best bit is, because pancakes can be sweet or savoury you can use berries, apples, bananas or even lemons, the pancake is your oyster (so to speak).

WHEAT GERM, BANANA & APPLE PANCAKES

Serves 4
Cooking Time: 20 minutes

INGREDIENTS

× 2 apples, peeled and diced
× 1 tablespoon unsalted butter
× ¼ teaspoon cinnamon
× 3 bananas
× 200 g (7 oz) buckwheat flour
× 50 g (13/4 oz) wheat germ
× 1 teaspoon baking powder

× 2 teaspoons sugar
× 1 teaspoon lemon juice
× 375 ml (13 fl oz) milk
× 1 egg
× 1 teaspoon vanilla extract
× maple syrup, to serve

METHOD

Place the diced apple in a mixing bowl and sprinkle with the cinnamon, tossing to coat well. Set aside.

Melt the butter and pour into a blender. Add the remaining ingredients (except the maple syrup) and purée till smooth. Pour the mixture over the apple mixture and stir to combine.

Place a non-stick frying pan over medium heat. Using a ladle, add the batter to the pan and cook until the batter starts to bubble and brown on the bottom, then flip over carefully.

When done, remove from the pan and cover with foil to keep warm. Repeat until all the batter is cooked. Serve warm with maple syrup.

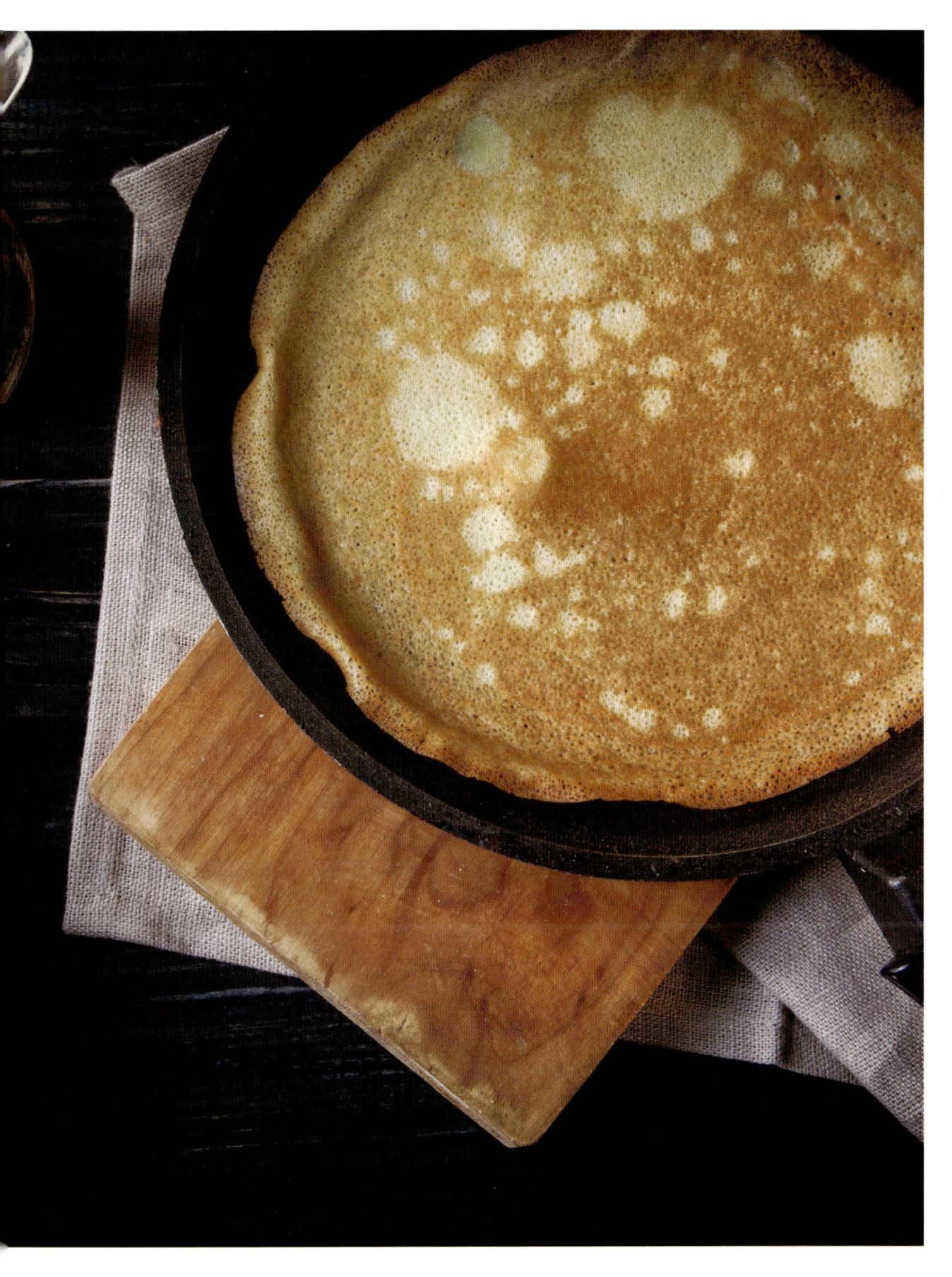

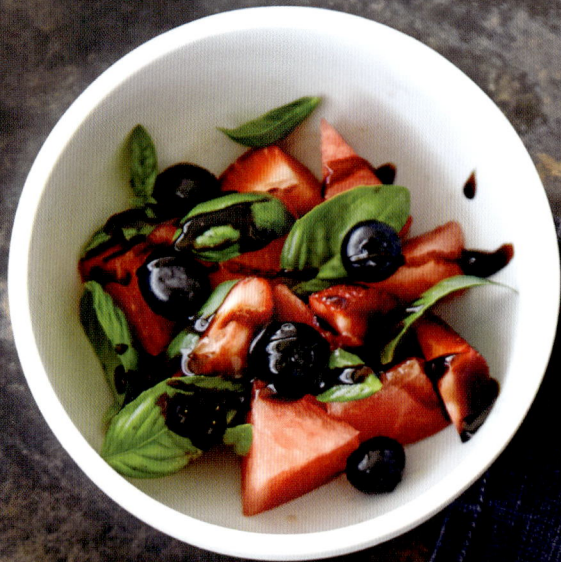

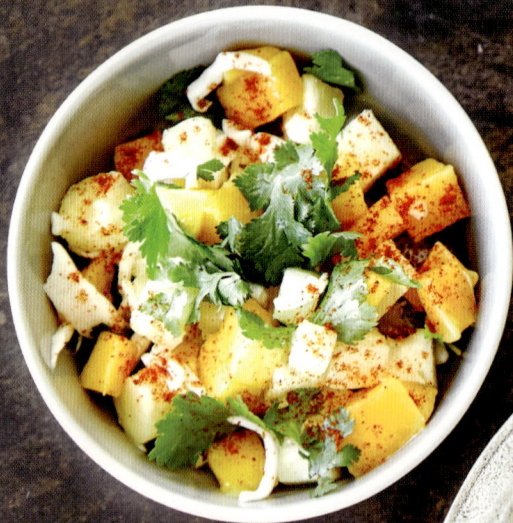

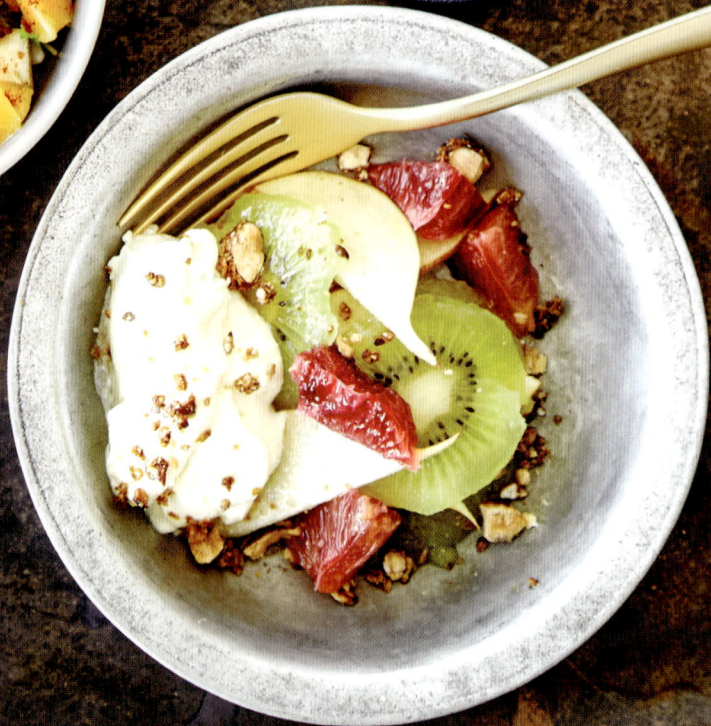

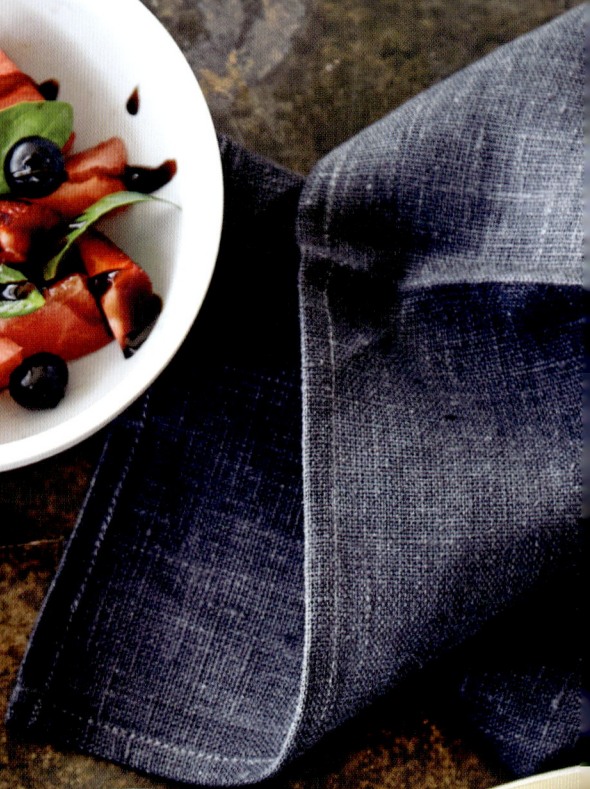

No matter what the season, fruit salad is a quick and easy way to make sure your partner has the fruits they need every day to stay healthy. But like anything else, the same old fruit salad day in and day out can get a little boring so here are some simple ideas you can use to mix up your fruit salads using nuts, herbs and even chilli to bring out a whole new dimension in flavour.

SUMMER FRUIT SALAD

Serves 4
Cooking Time: 5 minutes

INGREDIENTS

BALSAMIC HONEY GLAZE
× 3 tablespoons balsamic vinegar
× 1 tablespoon honey

× 300 g (10½ oz) watermelon, chopped into bite-sized pieces
× 200 g (7 oz) strawberries, hulled and quartered
× 100 g (3½ oz) blueberries
× 2 basil sprigs, leaves torn

METHOD

To make the balsamic honey glaze, combine the balsamic vinegar and honey in a bowl and set aside.
Add the watermelon, strawberries and blueberries to a mixing bowl.
Toss the basil leaves into the salad.
Drizzle over the balsamic honey glaze, gently toss again and serve immediately.

WINTER FRUIT SALAD

Serves 4
Cooking Time: 25 minutes

BURNT NUT CRUMBLE
- × 25 g (1 oz) hazelnut
- × 25 g (1 oz) pistachio nuts
- × 25 g (1 oz) almonds
- × 15 g (½ oz) wheat germ
- × 25 g (1 oz) puffed rice
- × 2 tablespoons molasses

- × 2 kiwi fruit, roughly chopped
- × 1 blood orange, roughly chopped
- × 2 nashi pear, roughly chopped
- × 2 tablespoons lime
- × 4 tablespoons Greek-style yoghurt

METHOD

Preheat the oven to 140°C (275°F/Gas 1). Line a baking tray with baking paper.

Process the hazelnuts, pistachio nuts and almonds in a food processor until they are roughly broken up. Transfer to a bowl.

Add the wheat germ and puffed rice to the nut mixture. Drizzle over the molasses, mixing well to ensure the ingredients are all coated.

Spread the nut mix over the baking paper. Place the tray in the oven and bake for 10 minutes, then move the mixture around on the paper. Bake for a further 5 minutes, then remove from the oven and allow to cool.

Add the kiwi fruit, blood orange and pear to a mixing bowl. Drizzle over the lime juice and gently toss together.

Serve the fruit in bowls with a generous amount of the burnt nut crumble sprinkled on top and a dollop of yoghurt.

This fruit salad is a variant on some of the incredible snacks you can pick up at street vendor stalls all along the Baja Peninsula in Mexico. The combination of the young coconut, lime, coriander and chilli is incredibly unique and makes for an unforgettable fruit salad. The chilli mix is mind-blowing if you can find all of the powders. If not, feel free to just sprinkle a combination of red chilli powder, salt and a touch of smoked paprika.

BAJA STREET VENDOR FRUIT SALAD

Serves 4
Cooking Time: 10 minutes

INGREDIENTS

STREET VENDOR CHILLI POWDER
- × ¼ red chilli powder
- × ¼ teaspoon chipotle chilli powder
- × ¼ teaspoon ancho chilli powder
- × ¼ teaspoon pasilla chilli powder
- × ¼ teaspoon mulato chilli powder
- × pinch of sea salt

- × 150 g (5½ oz) young coconut flesh, chopped
- × 150 g (5½ oz) pineapple, chopped
- × 200 g (7 oz) mango, chopped
- × ¼ bunch coriander (cilantro), roughly chopped
- × juice of 1/2 lime

METHOD

Place a small frying pan over low heat and add the red chilli, chipotle, ancho, pasilla and mulato chilli powder and salt. Cook until fragrant. Remove from the heat and set aside to cool.

Add the coconut flesh, pineapple, mango and coriander to a mixing bowl and gently toss to combine. Squeeze the lime juice over and toss the ingredients again.

To serve, simply add a portion of fruit to each bowl and sprinkle a tiny pinch of the street vendor chilli powder over the top.

Note: Store leftovers of the street vendor chilli powder in an airtight container for future use.

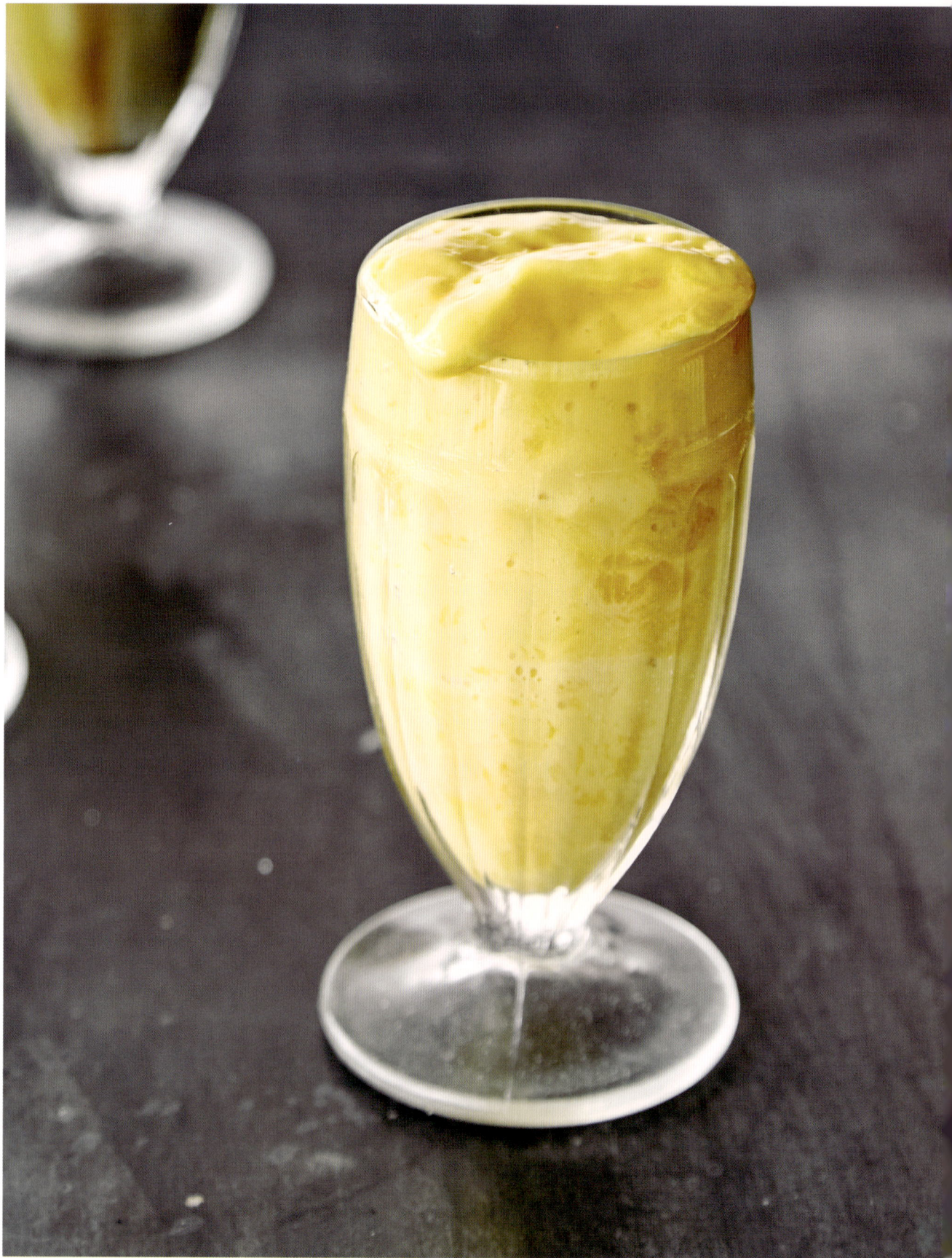

Shakes, smoothies or frappés, call them what you will but what they are is a glass packed full of goodness for your pregnant partner. I always like to include either a fruit or berry, some yoghurt and a grain in each glass but there really are no hard and fast rules, aside from tasting great.

BANANA SHAKE

Serves 4/Makes 1.25 litres (44 fl oz)
Cooking Time: 5 minutes

INGREDIENTS

- × 2 bananas, roughly chopped
- × 650 ml (221/2 fl oz) low-fat or skim milk
- × 2 tablespoons wheat germ
- × 6 tablespoons blueberry yoghurt
- × 1 tablespoon molasses

METHOD

Place the banana into a blender with the milk, wheat germ, blueberry yoghurt and molasses. Process in 10-second bursts until the mixture is smooth with no big lumps.
Serve cold with a meal or on its own as snack.

MANGO SHAKE

Makes 1.25 litres (44 fl oz)
Cooking Time: 5 minutes

INGREDIENTS

- × 200 g (7 oz) mango (frozen is fine if you can't get fresh), chopped
- × 325 ml (11 fl oz) low-fat or skim milk
- × 325 ml (11 fl oz) coconut water

- × 2 tablespoons almond meal
- × 6 tablespoons passionfruit yoghurt
- × 2 tablespoons honey

METHOD

Place the mango into a blender with the milk, coconut water, almond meal, passionfruit yoghurt and honey. Process in 10-second bursts until the mixture is smooth with no big lumps.

Serve cold with a meal or on its own as snack.

BLUEBERRY THICK SHAKE

Makes 1.25 litres (44 fl oz)
Cooking Time: 5 minutes

INGREDIENTS

- × 150 g (5 fl oz) blueberries
- × 650 ml (221/2 fl oz) low-fat or skim milk
- × 2 tablespoons buckwheat

- × 6 tablespoons date & coconut frozen yoghurt (see page 196)
- × 2 tablespoons maple syrup

METHOD

Place the blueberries, milk, buckwheat, yoghurt and maple syrup into a blender and process in 10-second bursts until the mixture is smooth with no big lumps.

Serve cold with a meal or on its own as snack.

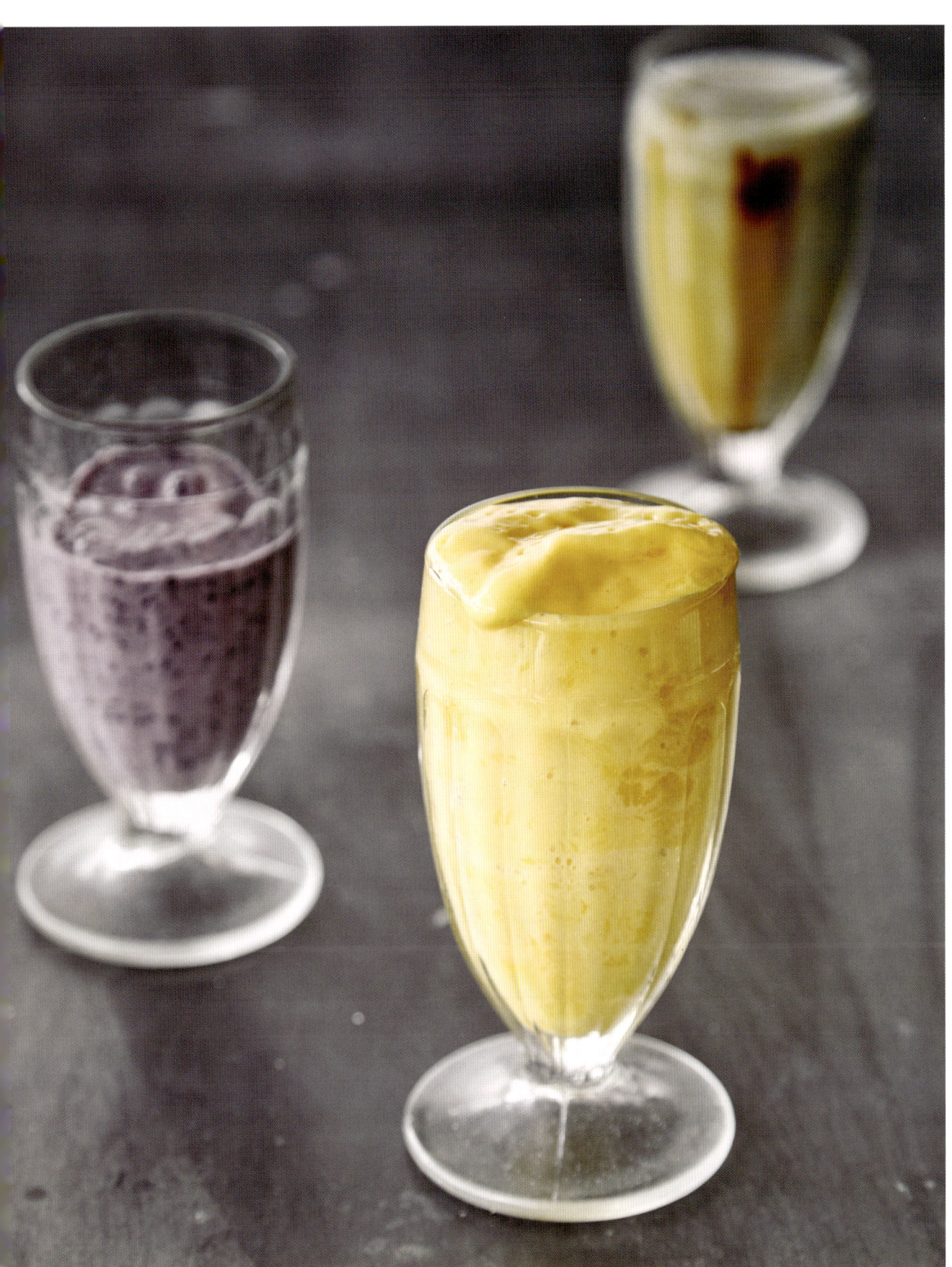

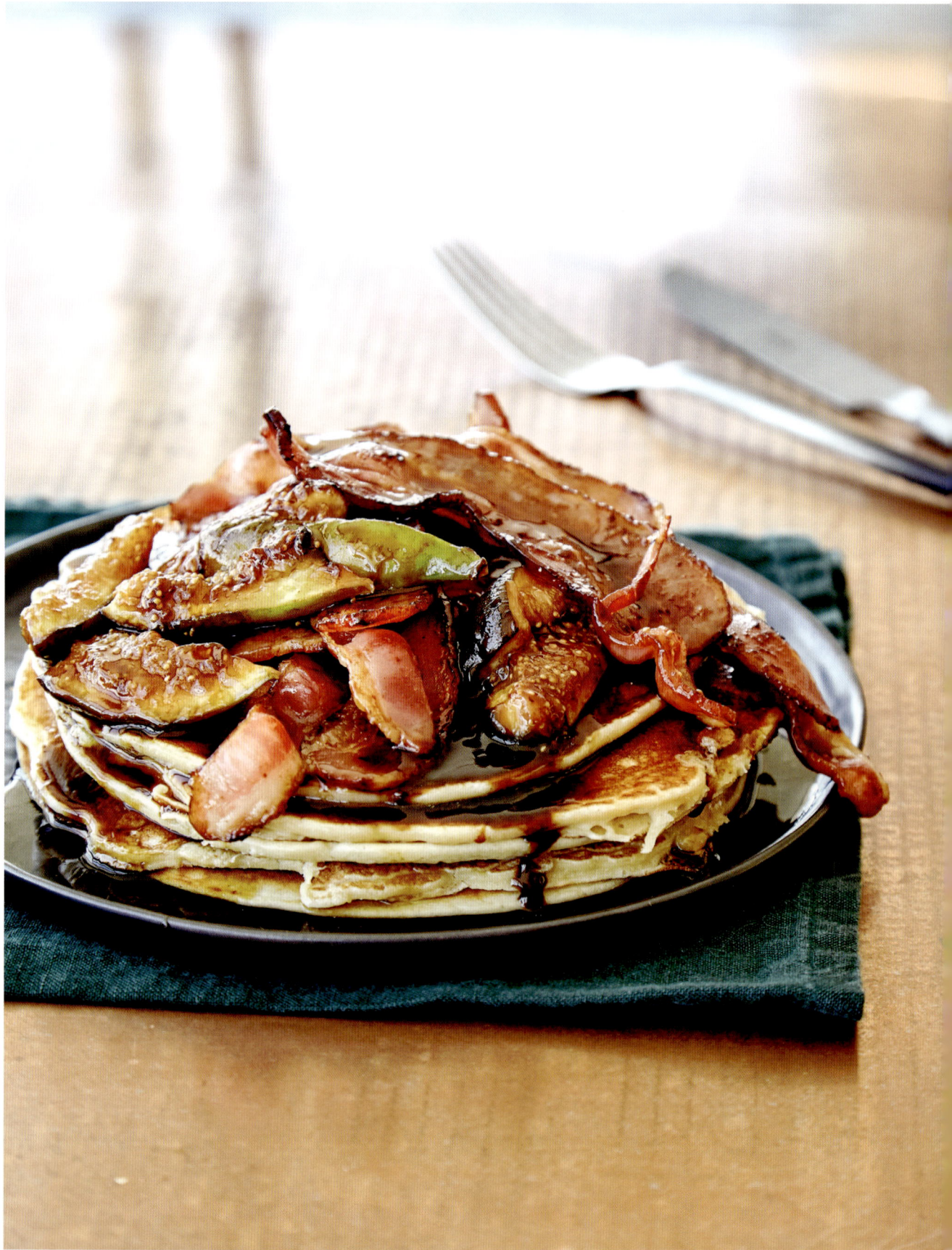

I have tried to include a variety of healthy options in this book; however, it would be remiss of me not to include some truly decadent recipes for those special days when you just want a delicious treat. This is one of my proudest creations and it is truly a sensory extravaganza. If you take the time on Sunday morning to make this over-the-top dish, I can promise you that you will be seduced by the dark flavours of burnt fig and maple syrup and teased by the salty goodness of bacon. In fact, it's so delicious that eggs may just stay off the Sunday breakfast menu for good.

BURNT FIG & BACON PANCAKES

Serves 4
Cooking Time: 30 minutes

INGREDIENTS

PANCAKES
- × 1 tablespoon unsalted butter, melted
- × 250 g (9 oz) plain (all-purpose) flour
- × 1 teaspoon baking powder
- × 2 tablespoons white sugar
- × ½ teaspoon salt
- × 375 ml (13 fl oz) milk
- × 2 eggs
- × 1 teaspoon vanilla extract

BURNT FIG & BACON
- × 1 tablespoon unsalted butter
- × 6 figs, quartered
- × 6 streaky bacon slices (I prefer hickory smoked), halved
- × 5 tablespoons maple syrup, plus extra to drizzle

METHOD

Preheat the oven to 50°C (122°F).

Melt the butter in a frying pan and pour into a blender. Add the flour, baking powder, sugar, salt, milk, eggs, vanilla extract to the blender and blend for 10 seconds, making sure that the ingredients are well mixed. If not, scrape any mixture stuck to the sides with a plastic spatula and blend again. The mixture should be pretty thick and not too runny so if you need to add a little more flour, feel free. Pour the mixture into a large bowl

Place a non-stick frying pan over medium heat. Ladle the mixture into the pan and move it around gently until you have the desired size pancake.

Continued⤵

BURNT FIG & BACON PANCAKES CONTINUED...

Cook until bubbles form in the batter and the underside is golden brown. Then flip over and cook until other side is golden. Remove from the pan, wrap it in foil and place in the oven to keep warm. Continue until the remaining batter is used.

Heat the butter in a non-stick frying pan over medium heat. Add the figs and fry until the fruit is dark, slightly burnt and soft. Remove and set aside.

Heat a splash of vegetable oil in the same frying pan over medium heat. Add the bacon and cook until lightly browned, then turn and repeat. Add the figs to the pan with the bacon. Reduce the heat to low and add the maple syrup to the pan, cooking until the sugar caramelizes and turns dark and shiny. Remove from the heat.

Remove the pancakes from the oven and stack on a serving plate. Spoon the fig and bacon mixture over the top, as well as the caramelised sauce. Cut the stack into quarters. Serve with more maple syrup to taste, if you like.

THE DISTANT MEMORY OF A GOOD NIGHT'S SLEEP

I feel like television might have lied to me when it comes to parenthood, and I feel a little betrayed.

At some point everyone has seen that episode in a TV show where they have the birth. You know the one, they rush to the hospital (where in-between the witty repartee in the waiting room and some crazy subplot involving a marriage proposal gone wrong or a mix up in the delivery room) and the lead actress finally brings her little bundle of joy into the world, without so much as breaking a heavy sweat. And when her perfect-looking newborn is placed into her arms, her brow still slightly damp and glistening beneath her perfectly tousled hair, the baby doesn't seem to cry at all, just coo and gurgle as the credits roll over a perfectly happy family.

So you can imagine my surprise when my little bundle of joy finally arrived a little more smooshed and purple looking than the groomed infant on the television. As the days went by I noticed that there were a lot of other things had been conveniently left until after the credits had rolled. Where were the endless nights of crying? The feeding frenzy, the infant acne, the farting, the thick coating of body hair or the endless stream of faeces that just seems to shoot out of babies' behinds with the force of a jumbo jet engine.

All of these things were cut out and left on the editing floor but unfortunately in real life nobody is going to give you a break when it all gets too much saying 'We'll be right back after these messages'.

Every expectant parent is painfully aware that they are about to face a marathon of sleepless nights but no matter what you do nothing can truly prepare you for the onslaught you will face those first few weeks when you get home from the hospital. As sleep deprivation is used as a form of torture in some countries, I found it a good idea to lighten the mood and have some fun. So why don't you try doing a couple of the activities that got me through those long, dark nights of crying.

Start keeping notes on how many hours your baby can cry in a day and then see if they can beat that record.

Find out which one of your friends 'hates it' when people fill up their social media stream with pictures of their newborn and then tag them in a flood of cutesy images.

Start making short films that always have a baby crying in the plot.

And if all else fails, start deliberately binge-watching terrible television shows. Who knows, after a couple of hours watching crazed bounty hunters, people fighting at storage container auctions or deluded housewives with too much plastic surgery, you may find you prefer the sound of a child screaming after all.

SOMETHING LIGHT

More than just the humble sandwich
(which amazingly contains several recipes for sandwiches)

From The Wise

One of the challenges of cooking for your pregnant partner is making sure you try and get as many servings from all of the required nutritional groups in every meal. Sandwiches are great for this as you can pack them full of all the good stuff and still leave room for a homemade shake or juice. This is an old school egg sandwich loaded up with rocket, spinach, cucumber and tarragon for a bit of zing.

EGG & CUCUMBER SANDWICH WITH SEEDED MUSTARD AND SPINACH

Serves 2
Cooking Time: 20 minutes

INGREDIENTS

- × 2 eggs
- × ½ tablespoon seeded mustard
- × 1 teaspoon tarragon, finely chopped
- × ½ tablespoon store-bought mayonnaise
- × 25 g (2 oz) rocket (arugula)
- × 25 g (2 oz) baby English spinach

- × 1 tablespoon olive oil
- × 1 teaspoon unsalted butter
- × 4 slices grain bread
- × 1 cucumber, thinly sliced
- × 10 g (½ oz) parmesan cheese, shaved
- × sea salt and cracked black pepper, to season

METHOD

Bring a small saucepan of water to a rolling boil and add the eggs. Cook the eggs until hard boiled (How long it takes to hard boil an egg really depends on the size and can range from between 10–15 minutes. If you are unsure then cook it for longer, it's going to be hard boiled anyway), then remove from the water. Peel the eggs and roughly chop.

Combine the mustard, chopped tarragon and mayonnaise in a small mixing bowl. Add the chopped egg and combine.

In another small mixing bowl, place the rocket and baby English spinach and toss with the olive oil. Season with salt and cracked black pepper.

Butter the bread on one side. Layer the cucumber, egg mix, shaved parmesan and the rocket and spinach on one slice of bread and top with the other slice. Repeat with remaining ingredients.

Serve with a Banana shake (page 67).

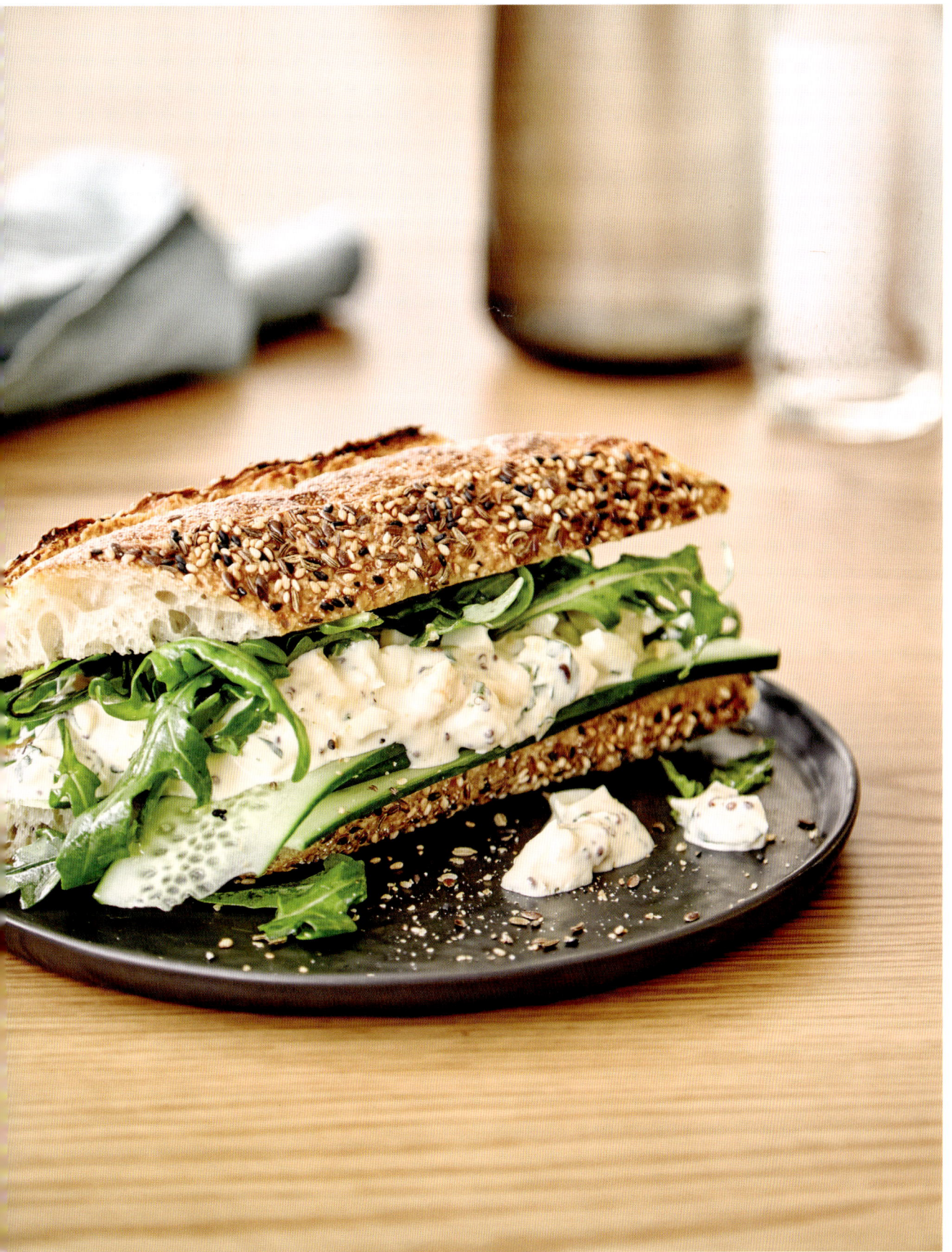

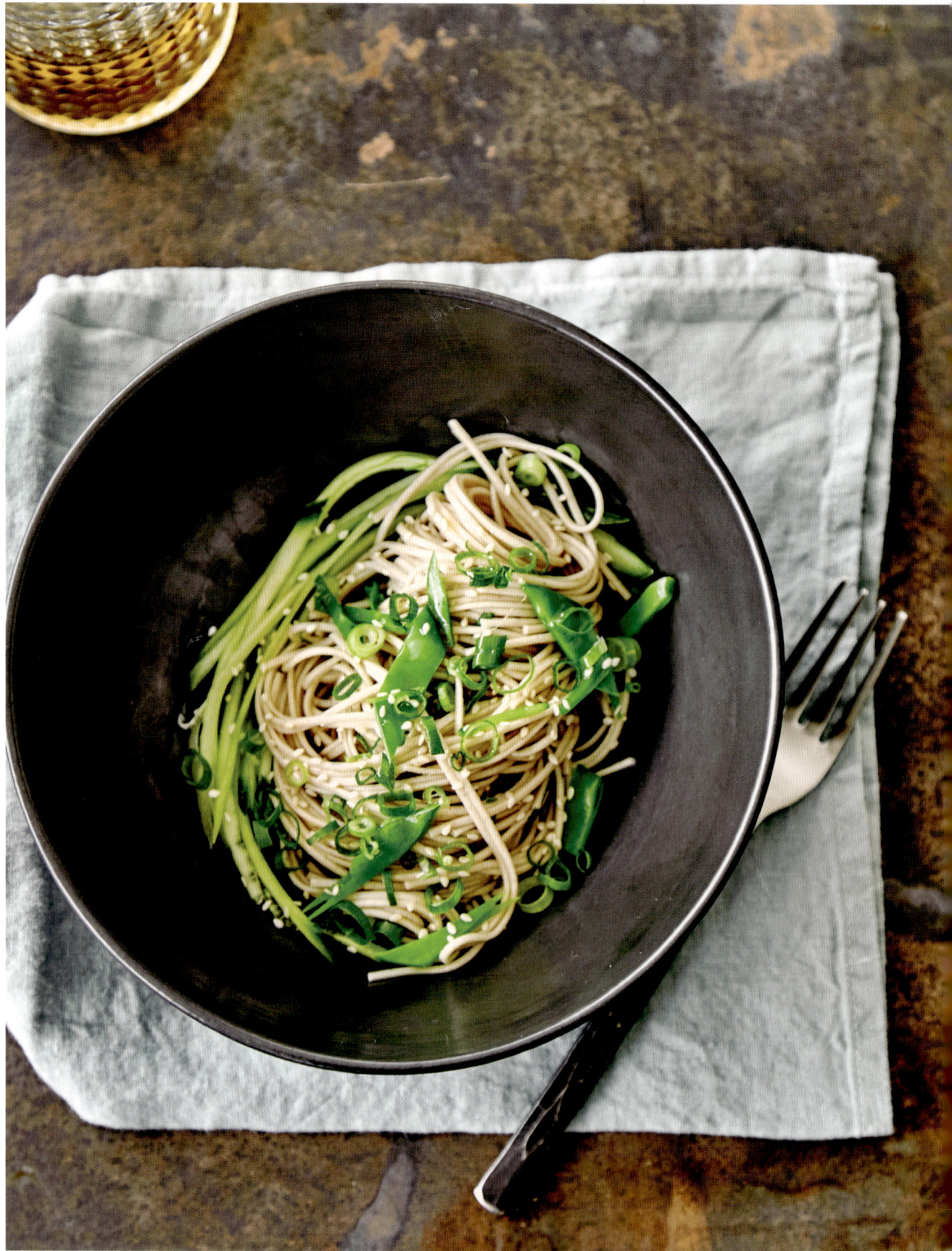

Cold soba noodle salad is a popular Japanese summertime dish that is normally served with the noodles in a bamboo basket and a dipping sauce on the side. I have added a couple of pregnancy-friendly ingredients to fortify the Japanese classic as well as combine the dipping sauce with the noodles to make it a little easier to eat.

SOBA NOODLE SALAD

Serves 4
Cooking Time: 30 minutes

INGREDIENTS

- × 2 tablespoons of rice wine vinegar
- × 50 ml (13/4 fl oz) light soy sauce
- × 1 teaspoon white sugar
- × ½ sachet dashi powder
- × 1 teaspoon sesame oil
- × 1 tablespoon sesame seeds
- × 150 g (51/2 oz) snow peas (mangetout), trimmed
- × 400 g (14 oz) soba noodles
- × 2 spring onion (scallion) stalks, thinly sliced
- × 1 Lebanese (short) cucumber, sliced lengthways into long, thin strips
- × 25 g (1 oz) ginger, peeled and julienned
- × 80 g (23/4 oz) baby English spinach, roughly chopped

METHOD

Place a large saucepan filled with water over medium heat and bring to the boil.

Using another saucepan, place over low heat and add the rice wine vinegar, light soy sauce, white sugar, dashi powder and sesame oil. Stir until sugar and dashi are dissolved, then remove from the heat and pour into a bowl, setting aside in the fridge to cool.

Place a dry frying pan over low heat and add the sesame seeds, toasting until fragrant. Remove from the heat and set aside.

Add the snow peas to a pot of boiling water and cook for 2 minutes. Place a colander in the sink and remove the snow peas from the water with tongs, then turn on the tap, running them under the cold water to cool.

Add the soba noodles to the boiling water and cook for 3 minutes. Remove the soba noodles from the water and rinse under the cold tap to cool. Drain for 5 minutes.

Place the noodles in a mixing bowl and add the spring onions, cucumber, ginger, snow peas and spinach, then drizzle the sauce mixture over the top, tossing together well.

Serve with a garnish of the sesame seeds on each plate.

This dish is a great example of the myriad of different types of salads you can whip up for a quick lunch or light dinner. The ingredients are interchangeable (I have used figs, pears, witlof and spinach) for whatever you might feel like or have on hand so don't feel like you have to stick to the recipe. You can add nuts or an egg, or change the fruit or the protein, it's up to you.

FIG, PEAR & PROSCIUTTO SALAD

Serves 4
Cooking Time: 20 minutes

INGREDIENTS

- × 150 g (51/2 oz) baby English spinach
- × 6 white witlof (chicory/Belgian endive) heads
- × 1 nashi pear, quartered and thinly sliced
- × 10 g (½ oz) parmesan cheese, grated
- × 1 pomegranate
- × 8 figs, quartered
- × 1 tablespoon balsamic vinegar glaze
- × 12 prosciutto slices
- × 4 tablespoons olive oil
- × sea salt and cracked black pepper, to season

METHOD

Add the spinach, witlof and pear to a mixing bowl. Grate over the parmesan cheese.

Cut the pomegranate in half and squeeze the seeds over the salad.

Place a frying pan over medium heat and drizzle with some olive oil. Add the figs, cooking until browned. Add the balsamic vinegar and toss well. Remove the figs from the heat and set aside on a plate.

Wipe the pan clean and place back over medium heat, add some olive oil and the prosciutto. Fry the prosciutto until crispy on both sides, then remove from heat. Leave to cool slightly, then roughly chop and drain on a paper towel.

Add the figs and the prosciutto to the salad. Dress with olive oil and season with sea salt and cracked black pepper. Gently toss together and serve while the prosciutto is warm.

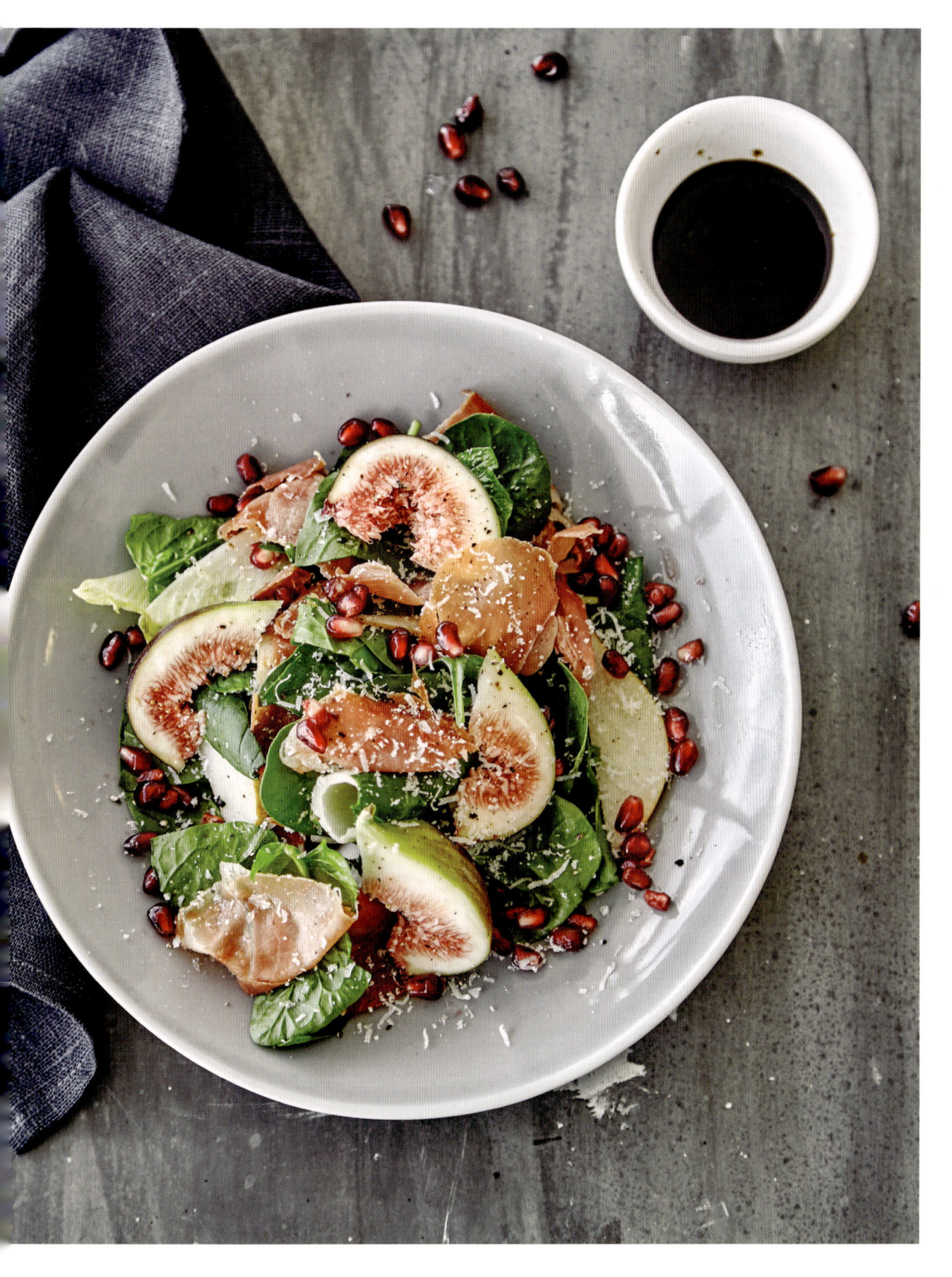

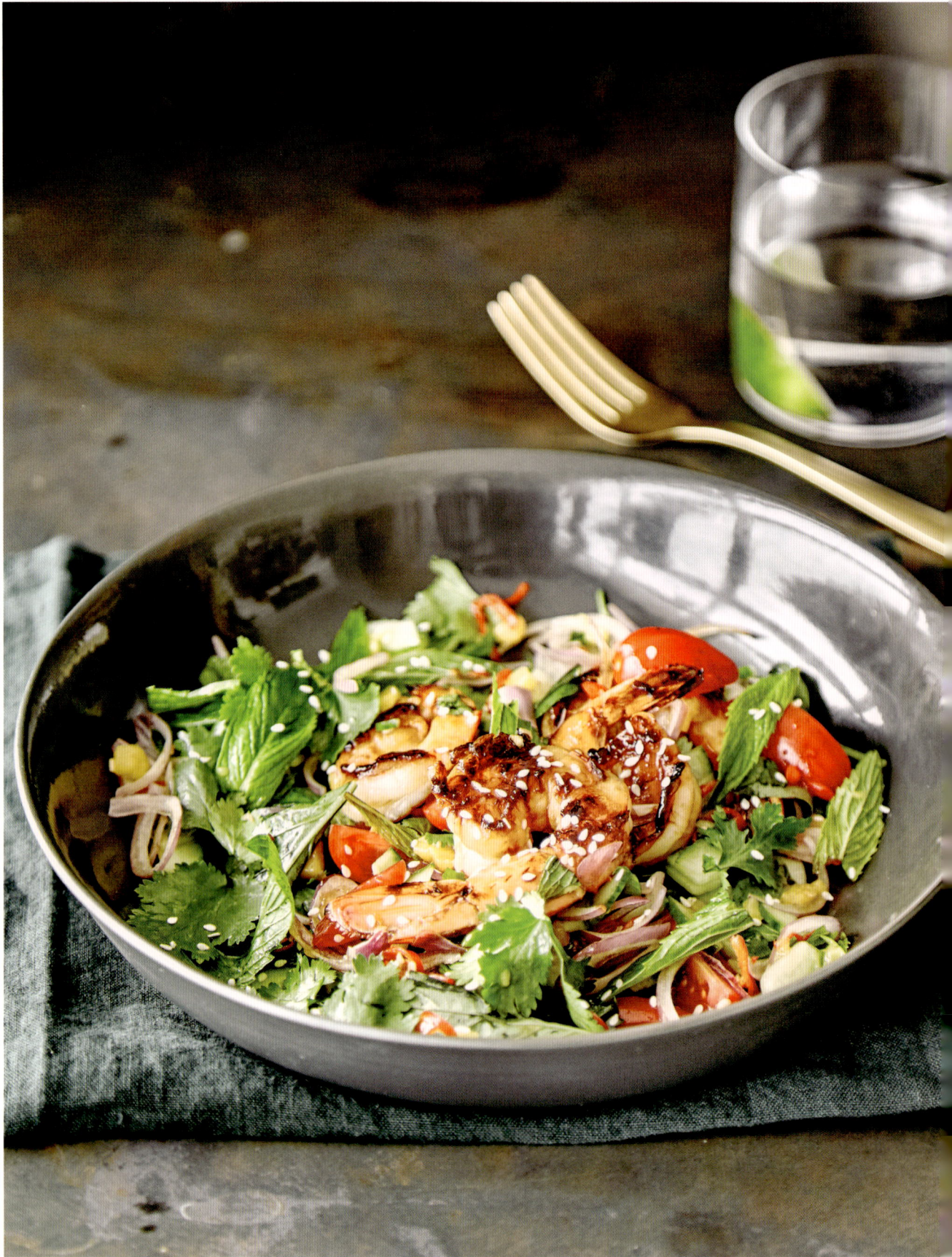

Sometimes you want to make something that's quick, easy, has close to twenty different ingredients in it and tastes great. If that's what you're in the mood for then this is definitely the dish for you. The beauty of this dish is that the protein is easily substituted; prawns make them feel queasy—no problem, just swap it out for some calamari. Not eating enough red meat, ditch the mango and add some thinly sliced flank steak.

PRAWN/SHRIMP & MANGO SALAD

Serves 4
Cooking Time: 20 minutes

INGREDEIENTS

PRAWN/SHRIMP & MANGO SALAD
- ½ bunch mint leaves, roughly torn
- ½ bunch coriander (cilantro) leaves, roughly torn
- ½ bunch Thai basil leaves, roughly torn
- 4 red chillies, deseeded, thinly sliced (optional)
- ¼ red onion, thinly sliced
- 1 spring onion (scallion) stalk, thinly sliced
- ½ mango, diced
- 1 continental (long) cucumber, diced
- 10 cherry tomatoes, halved
- 12 prawns (shrimp), peeled and deveined
- 1 tablespoon sesame seeds, to garnish

DRESSING
- 1 garlic clove, crushed
- 15 g (½ oz) fresh ginger, finely chopped
- 2 teaspoons palm sugar
- 2 tablespoons fish sauce
- 2 tablespoons grapeseed oil
- ½ lime

METHOD

Place the mint, coriander and Thai basil in a large bowl. Add the chillies, onion and spring onion and mix to combine. Add the mango, cucumber and tomatoes and gently mix to combine. Preheat a barbecue hotplate or chargrill pan to medium heat.

Using a mortar and pestle, crush the garlic, ginger and palm sugar into a paste. Add the fish sauce, grapeseed oil and lime juice, mixing together well (if you don't have a mortar and pestle you can use a food processor). Taste the dressing to check there is a balance between salty and sweet, adding more salt or sugar if required.

Place the prawns/shrimp on the hot barbecue or chargrill pan and grill until fully cooked through on both sides. (No raw seafood for pregnant mothers, so cut one in half to make sure it is cooked through.).

Add the dressing to the salad and toss together well. Place the salad onto each plate and dress with three prawns, garnishing with sesame seeds.

This simple soup of prawns, udon noodles, mushrooms and spinach is a excellent dish to have in your arsenal as it tastes great, is not too harsh or heavy for an upset stomach and there are lots of different versions you can make. For something quick and easy, you could ditch the prawns and add a boiled egg or, for something a little more decadent, you could add some Karaage chicken (page 107).

POACHED PRAWN UDON NOODLE SOUP

Serves 4
Cooking Time: 35 minutes

INGREDIENTS

- × 6 dried shiitake mushrooms
- × 2 sachets instant dashi powder
- × 3 tablespoons light soy sauce
- × 2 tablespoons of rice wine vinegar
- × 12 prawns (shrimp), peeled and deveined

- × 250 g (9 oz) udon noodles
- × 100 g (31/2 oz) baby English spinach leaves
- × 25 g (1 oz) fresh peeled ginger, julienned
- × 1 spring onion (scallion) stalk, finely chopped

METHOD

Add the mushrooms to a small bowl and submerge in 125 ml (4 fl oz) of warm water, soaking for about 15 minutes (if mushrooms float to the surface weigh them down with a can or bowl.) Remove the mushrooms from the water (don't throw the soaking liquid out, we're going to use it) and thinly slice. Put the mushrooms and liquid aside.

Pour 750 ml (26 fl oz) of water into a saucepan over high heat and bring to the boil. Add the dashi powder, soy, rice wine vinegar and the liquid the mushrooms were soaked in and reduce to a simmer.

Add the prawns to the saucepan and cook for about 8 minutes, or until fully cooked through.

Add the shiitake mushrooms, udon noodles and spinach and cook for about 2 minutes.

To serve, place the udon noodles and three prawns in each bowl, using tongs, and then ladle the soup and spinach over the top, garnishing with the ginger and spring onions.

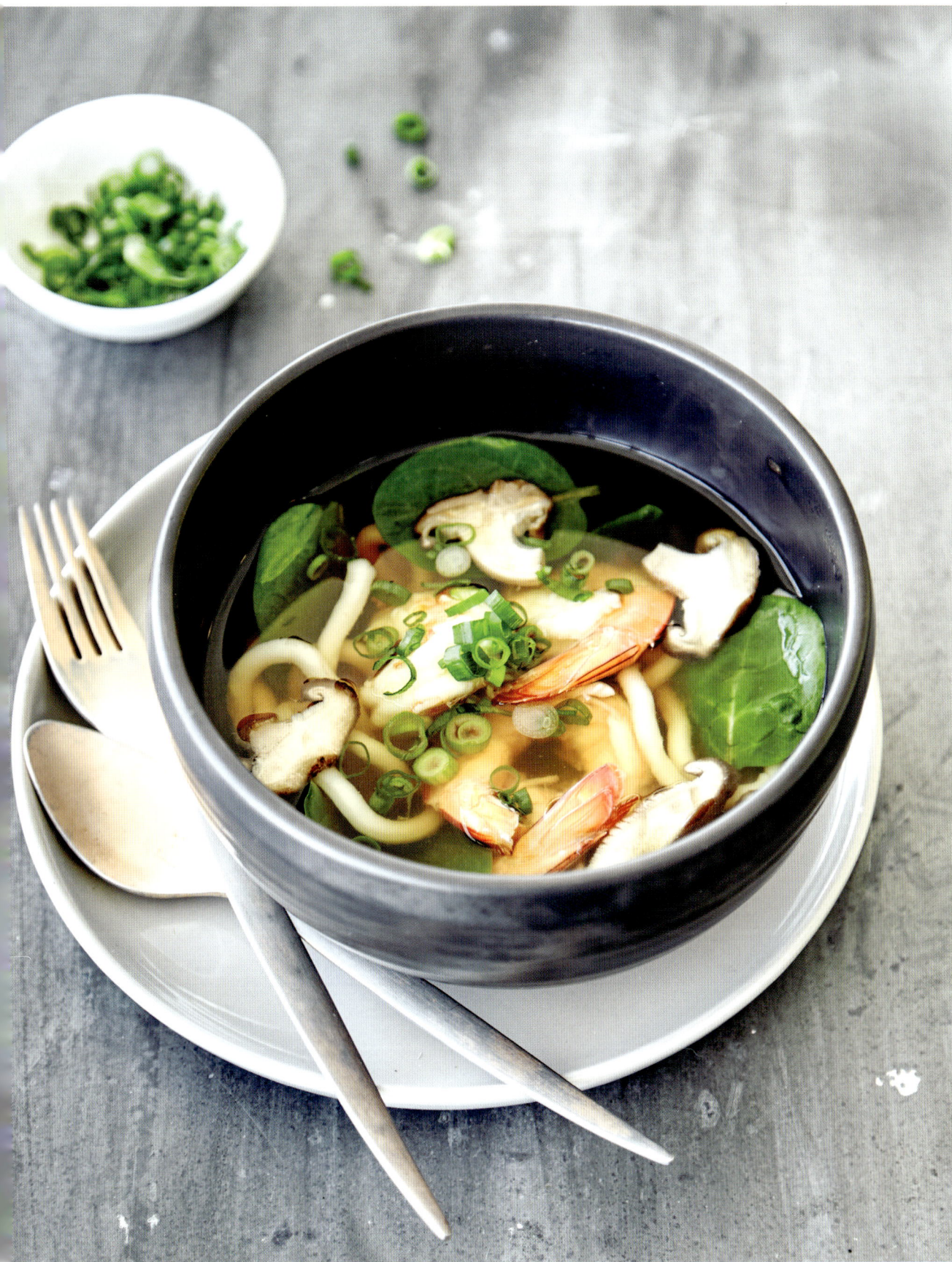

There are these humble, hole-in-the-wall sandwich shops that are scattered across the suburbs of most cities like hidden gems, from the outside appearing to be nothing more than a simple Vietnamese bakery. And to the uninitiated, I am sure it is confusing when they see lines fifty people deep outside these little stores at lunch time every single day. That is unless you've had a Bánh mì before and understand just how knee-bucklingly delicious they are. Unfortunately for expectant mothers though they are a big no-go during pregnancy so I have come up with a homemade, pregnancy-friendly version for you to make. Drop the mushroom pâté if you just want to make something quick, but if your partner is a fan you will win many brownie points when you put this on the table at lunchtime.

CARAMELIZED CHICKEN BÁNH MÌ WITH MUSHROOM PÂTÉ

Serves 4
Cooking Time: 45 minutes

INGREDIENTS

PICKLED CARROT
× 2 tablespoons brown sugar
× 3 tablespoons white vinegar
× 4 tablespoons fish sauce
× 2 carrots, grated

CARAMELIZED CHICKEN
× 4 chicken thighs
× 4 tablespoons kecap manis
× 15 g (½ oz) fresh ginger, grated
× 2 garlic cloves, crushed

MUSHROOM PÂTÉ
× 30 ml (1 fl oz) olive oil
× 1½ tablespoons butter
× 400 g (14 oz) mushrooms (I used shiitake and

portabella), finely chopped
× 2 brown shallots, diced
× 6 thyme sprigs, finely chopped
× 3 parsley sprigs, finely chopped
× sea salt and cracked black pepper, to season
× 30 ml (2 fl oz) white wine vinegar
× 3 tablespoons chicken stock (see Basics, page 31 or use unsalted if store-bought)

× 4 white, super fresh and crunchy baguettes
× 4 tablespoons store-bought mayonnaise
× 1 cucumber, finely sliced lengthways
× a dash of Maggi seasoning sauce (or soy sauce)
× 4 red Thai chillies (optional), finely sliced
× ½ bunch coriander (cilantro), chopped
× chilli sauce (optional)

To make the pickled carrot, place the sugar, vinegar and fish sauce into a mixing bowl and combine. Add the grated carrot into the bowl and mix to combine. Refrigerate for 30 minutes.

To make the caramelized chicken, place the chicken thighs in a mixing bowl and add the kecap manis, ginger and garlic and mix well. Refrigerate for 30 minutes to marinate.

To make the mushroom pâté, heat the oil and butter in a non-stick frying pan over medium heat. Add the mushrooms, shallots, thyme and parsley, then season with salt and cracked black pepper and cook until browned on all sides. Add the white wine vinegar and reduce by half, then add the chicken stock and cook until fully reduced. Remove from the heat and leave to cool slightly. Place the mixture in a food processor and blend until smooth. Transfer to an airtight container and store in the fridge.

Heat the vegetable oil in a large non-stick frying pan over medium heat. Add the chicken and cook until sticky and caramelized on one side, then flip over and repeat. Check to see the chicken is cooked through (cut one in half), then remove from the heat and cut up into bite-sized pieces.

Cut the baguettes in half and slather one side with mayonnaise and the other in the mushroom pâté. Top with the cucumber slices. Squeeze any excess liquid from the pickled carrot so they are moist but not soaking and place on top of the cucumber. Add the chicken to each baguette. Season generously with the Maggi seasoning and top with Thai chillies and coriander and, for those who like it extra hot, some chilli sauce. Serve immediately.

Funtastic Baby Facts.
Did you know a newborn needs to be fed anywhere from eight to twelve times a day?

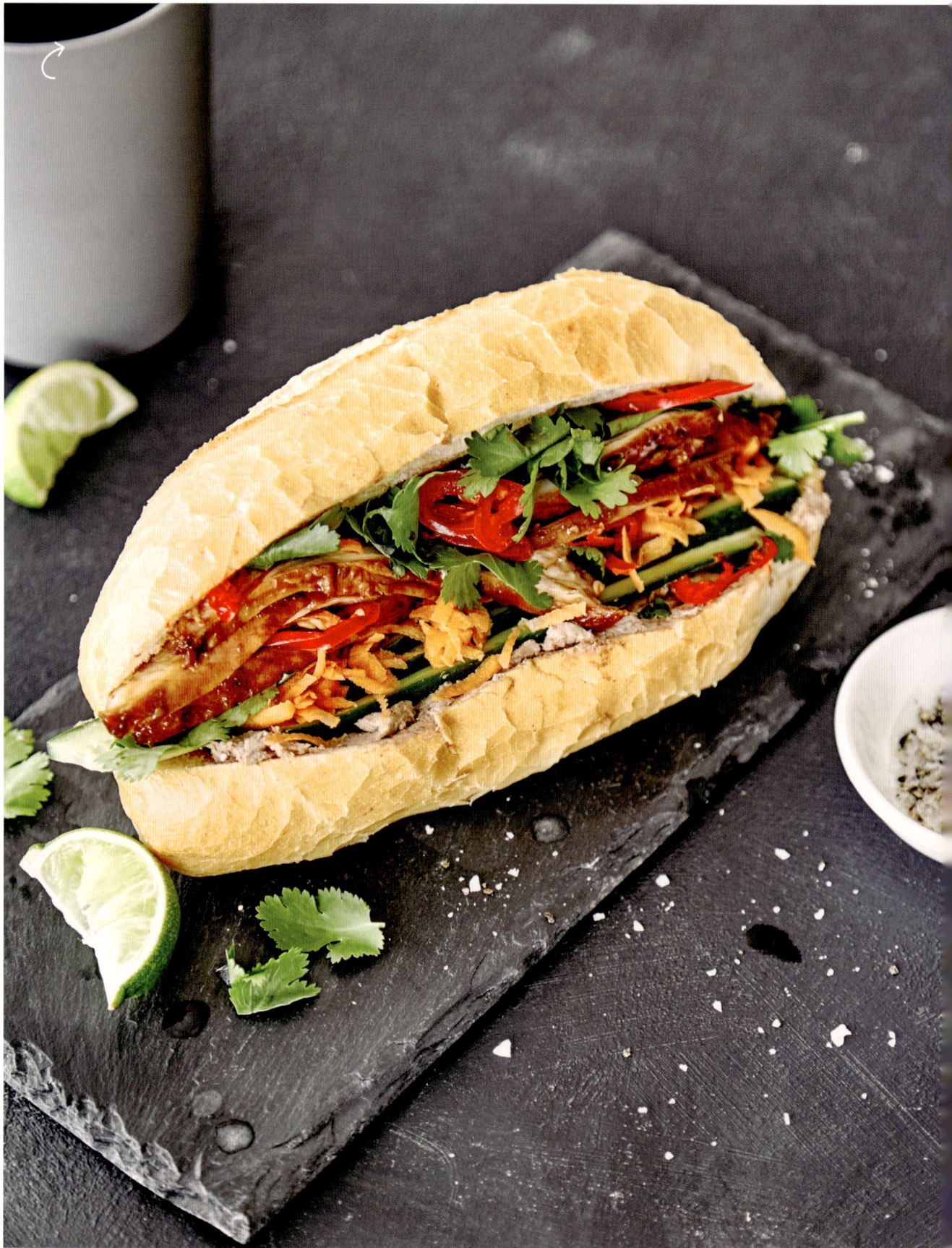

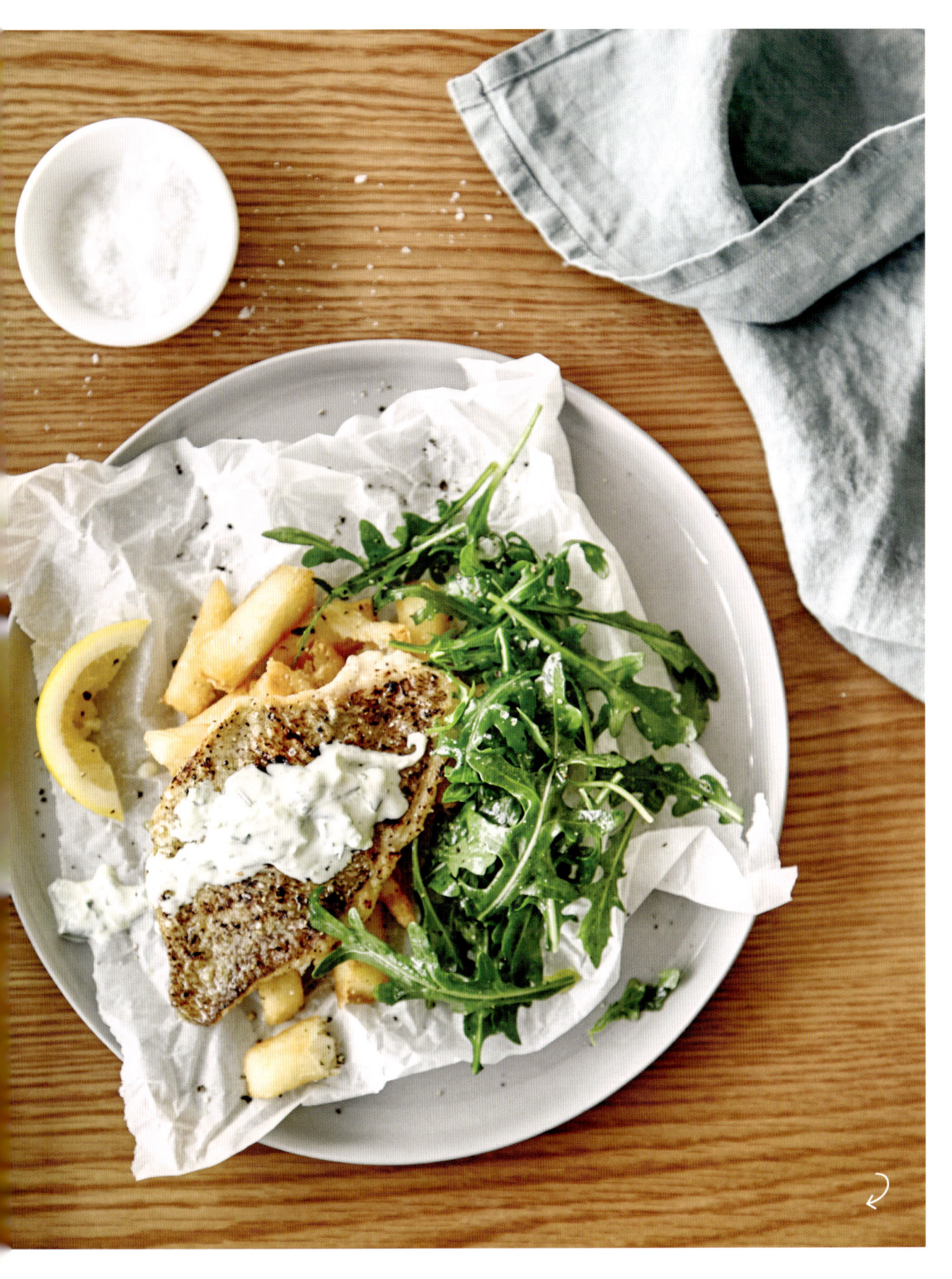

Now don't get me wrong, I love fish and chips as much as the next person but they can be a little on the greasy side. So this is a healthier version of the classic, with grilled fish, baked chips and a yoghurt-based tartare sauce.

FISH N' CHIPS

Serves 4

Cooking Time: 45 minutes.

INGREDIENTS

× 2 large potatoes, peeled and cut into thick chips
× 3 tablespoons olive oil, plus extra for drizzling
× 3 tablespoons plain (all-purpose) flour
× 4 fillets snapper (scaled, with skin on)
× sea salt and cracked black pepper, to season
× ¼ bunch flat-leaf (Italian) parsley, roughly chopped, to garnish

YOGURT TARTARE SAUCE
× 130 g (4½ oz) Greek-style yoghurt
× 1 pickled cucumber, chopped
× 1 tablespoon pickled cucumber brine/vinegar
× ¼ bunch dill, roughly chopped
× 1 teaspoon capers
× 1 lemon, quartered

METHOD

Fill a large saucepan two-thirds full with salted water and bring to boil over medium heat.

Add the chips to the boiling water and cook for about 10 minutes (fork should enter without resistance). Carefully remove from the boiling water using a slotted spoon and place in a colander to drain for 1 minute.

Meanwhile, make the yoghurt tartare sauce. Place the yoghurt, pickled cucumber, brine, dill and capers in a food processor. Squeeze a lemon quarter into the food processor and season with sea salt and cracked black pepper. Process until the ingredients are combined. Remove the mixture from the processor and store in an airtight container in the fridge until needed.

Heat the oven grill (broiler) to high. Lightly grease a baking tray with olive oil.

Place the chips in a large bowl and poke them with a fork to break them up. Drizzle over 3 tablespoons of the olive oil and toss to coat well. Lay the chips out on the baking tray (the broken fluffy parts are going to turn into delicious crunchy brown bits so it's fine if a few of them break apart).

Place the tray under the oven grill (broiler) and cook until golden brown (remember to move them around so all sides get cooked properly). When finished, remove the tray from the oven and place the chips in a bowl lined with paper towels to remove any excess oil. Season with sea salt.

Add the flour to a large plate. Pat the fish dry with paper towel, then place skin side down in the flour to coat, shaking off any excess.

Heat the olive oil in a frying pan over medium heat. When hot, add the fish skin side down. Press the fish down firmly against the pan once to ensure it is getting even contact with the heat and leave to cook without turning until the skin is golden brown. Carefully turn the fish over and cook for 2–3 minutes on the other side (check to see the fish is fully cooked through) and remove from the pan.

To serve, place a piece of fish on each plate, top with a generous squeeze of the remaining lemon and season with sea salt and cracked black pepper. Garnish with some parsley. Add the chips, with a tablespoon of the tartare sauce. Serve with one of the Simple Salads (page 103-106).

From The Wise

The key to this recipe is the size of the mushrooms and the broccoli. Although it is a little time-consuming to dice everything before cooking it, the idea is that the mushrooms and broccoli will clump together inside the tiny shells of pasta. However, if you are time poor and not in the mood to stand in the kitchen for half an hour, feel free to roughly chop everything and throw it in the pan.

ORECCHIETTE WITH BROCCOLI AND PAN FRIED MUSHROOMS

Serves 4
Cooking Time: 30 minutes

INGREDIENTS

× 400g (14 oz) mushrooms, diced
× 200g (7 oz) broccoli, chopped
× 400g (14 oz) orecchiette pasta
× 4 tablespoons olive oil, plus extra for frying
× 2 tablespoons unsalted butter
× 2 garlic cloves, finely chopped

× 1 tablespoon dried chilli flakes (optional)
× ½ lemon, halved, seeds removed
× sea salt and cracked black pepper, to season
× 40 g (1½ oz) parmesan cheese, grated
× continental parsley, to garnish

METHOD

Heat a drizzle olive oil in a non-stick frying pan over medium heat. When hot, add the mushrooms (be careful not to overcrowd the pan. Cook in two batches if necessary as mushrooms have a tendency to sweat when crowded). Cook the mushrooms until browned on all sides, then remove from the heat and set aside in a bowl.

Return the frying pan to the cooktop and drizzle with olive oil. Add the broccoli and cook until tender, then add to the bowl with the mushrooms. Set aside.

Bring a saucepan of salted water to the boil. Carefully pour the pasta into the boiling salted water and cook until *al dente*. Remove from the heat and drain pasta (save a couple of tablespoons of the starchy pasta water).

Heat the olive oil and butter in a large non-stick frying pan over medium heat. Add the garlic and the dried chilli and stir. Add the mushrooms, broccoli and pasta water and stir.

Add the pasta to the pan and combine well, tossing or stirring the pasta and making sure all the tasty goodness from the bottom of the pan is distributed throughout the pasta.

Use a fork to squeeze out the lemon juice over the pasta. Season with sea salt and cracked black pepper to taste, tossing or stirring the pasta one last time.

Serve with the grated parmesan cheese and garnish with parsley. Serve with one of the Simple Salads (see page 103-106).

Funtastic Baby Facts

Did you know most babies double their birth weight by six months? Thankfully they slow down a little after that.

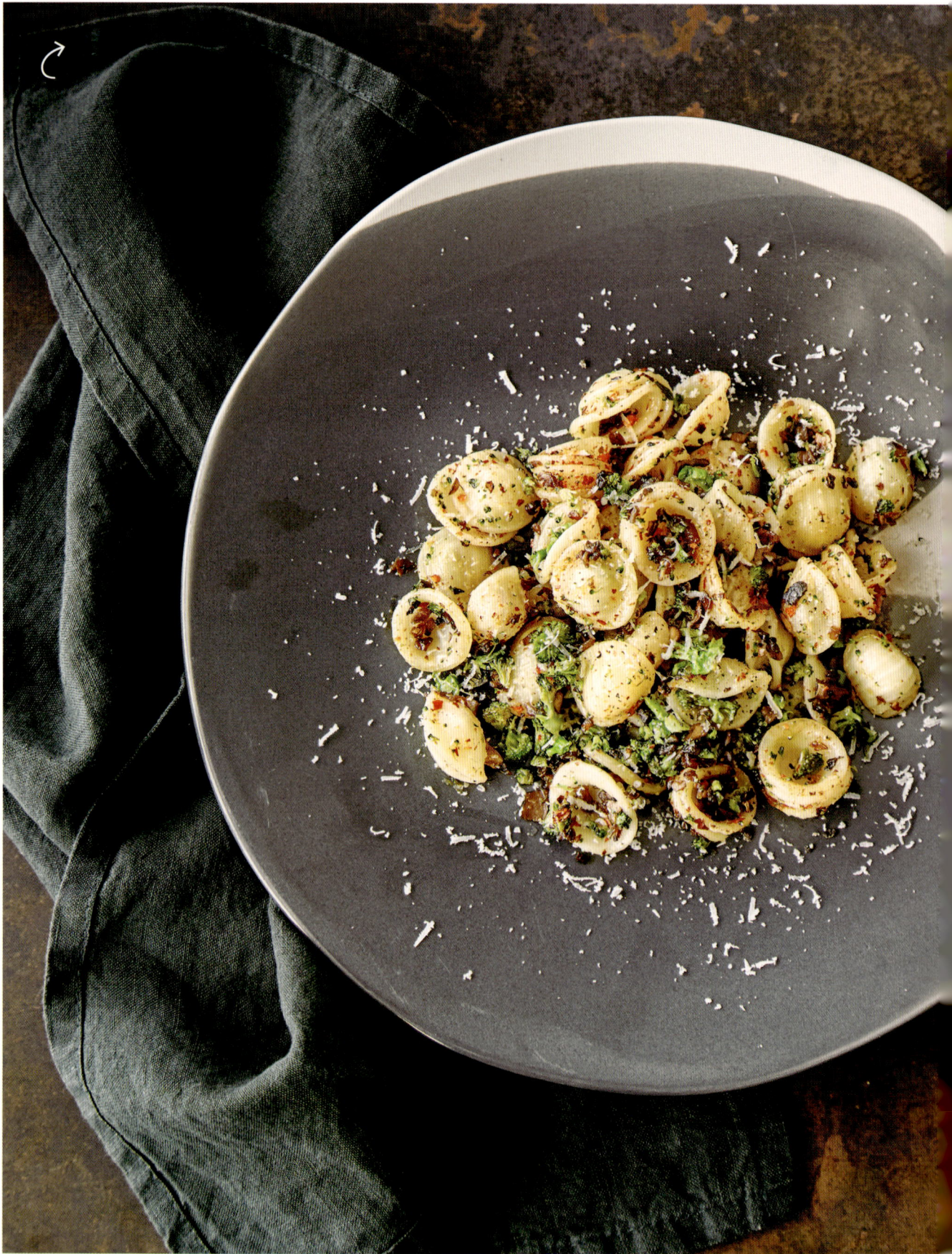

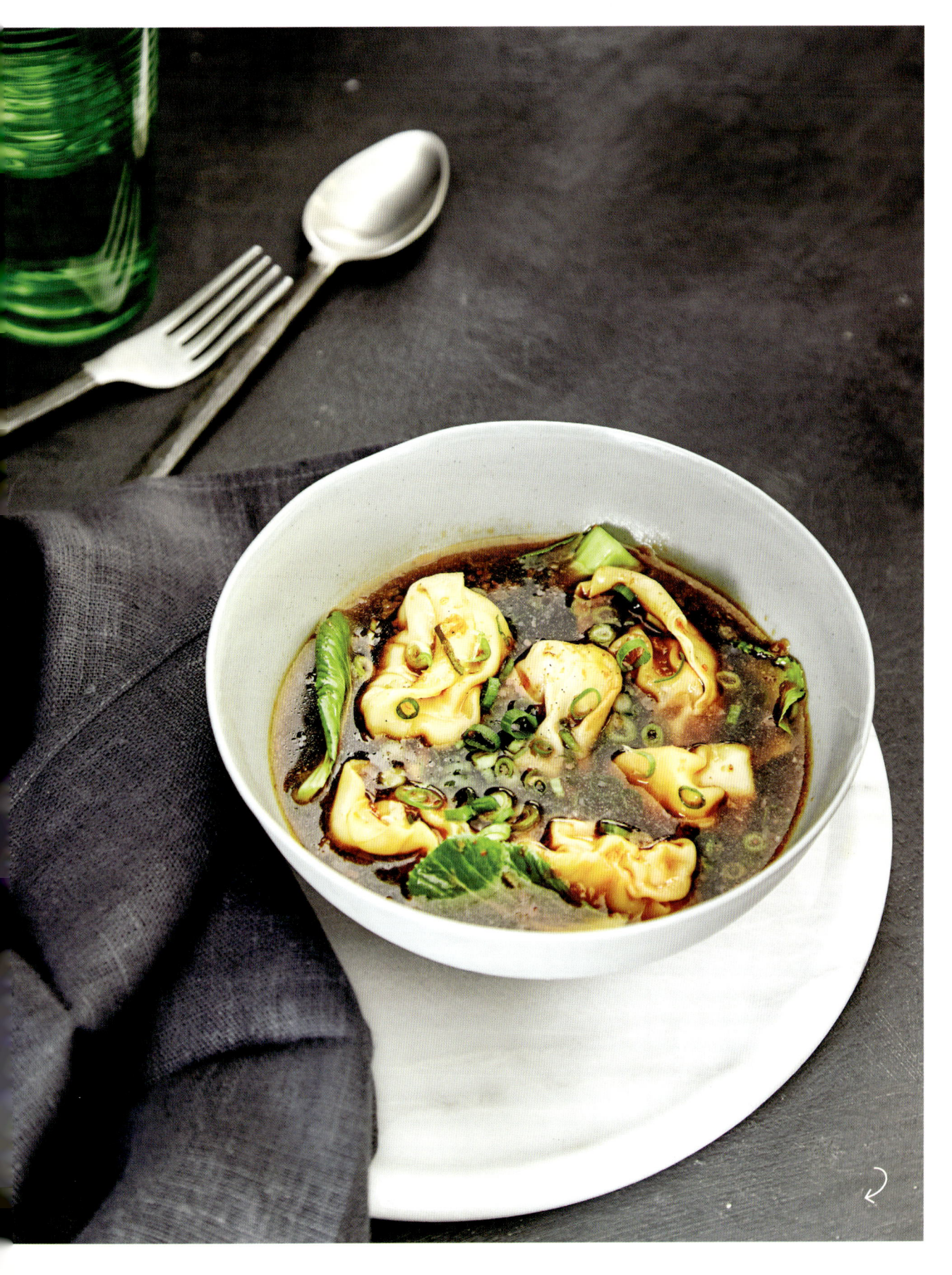

To me there was always one good reason to drag yourself out of bed on a Sunday and that was yum cha. Then I became a Dad and now have no choice but to be dragged out of bed early regardless what day of the week it is.

Going to yum cha is always a sensory overload. You're tempted by the exotic, mouthwatering delights that issue from the teetering towers of bamboo steamers, stacked high upon the shambolic jalopies careening their way through the crowded restaurant with an energy totally uncharacteristic for a lazy Sunday.

If you can't get away for yum cha but still have the taste for dumplings, these spicy Sichuan chilli wontons are great to make for lunch on a Sunday. I have used pork in the filling but feel free to mix it up and use vegetable, prawn, scallop or chicken.

SPICY SICHUAN PORK & CHIVE WONTONS

Serves 6
Cooking Time: 1 hour 20 minutes

INGREDIENTS

CHILLI OIL

× 150 ml (5 fl oz) peanut oil
× 25 g (1 oz) ground chilli flakes
× 25 g (1 oz) fresh ginger, julienned
× 3 garlic cloves, crushed

PORK & CHIVE WONTON

× ½ bunch chives, finely chopped
× 500g (17½ oz) minced (ground) pork
× 4 tablespoons light soy sauce
× 1 packet square wonton wrappers

SICHUAN PEPPER STOCK

× 20 Sichuan peppercorns
× 1 tablespoon peanut oil
× 25 g (1 oz) fresh ginger, julienned
× 4 garlic cloves, crushed
× 2 spring onions (scallions), finely sliced
× 4 shallots, finely chopped
× 500 ml (17 fl oz) chicken stock (see Basics, page 31 or use unsalted if store-bought)
× 3 tablespoons Chinese black vinegar
× 2 tablespoons light soy sauce
× 2 tablespoons caster (superfine) sugar
× 1 teaspoon sea salt
× 2 tablespoons chilli oil
× 1 bunch bok choy (pak choy), roughly chopped

To make the chilli oil, heat the peanut oil in a saucepan over low heat. Add the chilli flakes (sieve through small colander to remove the seeds if you want to control the heat), ginger and garlic to the pan. Cook until the oil starts to bubble, then remove from the heat and allow to cool. Store in an airtight container and set aside.

To make the wontons, add the chives to a mixing bowl. Add the minced pork and soy sauce and mix to combine.

Fill a small bowl with water. Line a tray with baking paper. Grab a wonton wrapper and dip your finger in the water, tracing around the edges so they are wet.

Add 1 teaspoon of pork mixture to the centre of the wrapper and fold over itself to make a rectangle, with the filling on the side closest to you, making sure that the air has been pressed out and the edges are sealed. Bring the bottom corners of wonton wrapper together over the mixture and pinch to secure leaving the top unfolded. Place the wonton on the baking tray.

Repeat until all of the meat has been used, ensuring the wontons are well spaced out on the tray and refrigerate for later.

To make the Sichuan pepper stock, place a small frying pan over low heat and add the Sichuan peppercorns, cooking until fragrant. Remove from the heat and crush using a mortar and pestle or a rolling pin.

Heat the peanut oil in a saucepan over low heat. Add the ginger, garlic, spring onions, shallots and Sichuan peppers and cook until fragrant. Increase the heat to medium and add the chicken stock, vinegar, soy sauce, sugar, salt and stir well. Bring to the boil, then reduce the heat to a low simmer. Cover and cook for 20 minutes. Remove the lid and reduce for further 10 minutes.

Add 2 heaped tablespoons of the chilli oil to the broth (the amount is optional depending on pregnant partner's tolerance of chilli). Add the bok choy and the pork and chive wontons to the broth and cook for a further 8–10 minutes (check a wonton before serving by cutting in half to make sure it is fully cooked). Season to taste.

Carefully scoop out the wontons and place them in a large serving bowl. Pour the stock mixture over the top and garnish with spring onions to serve.

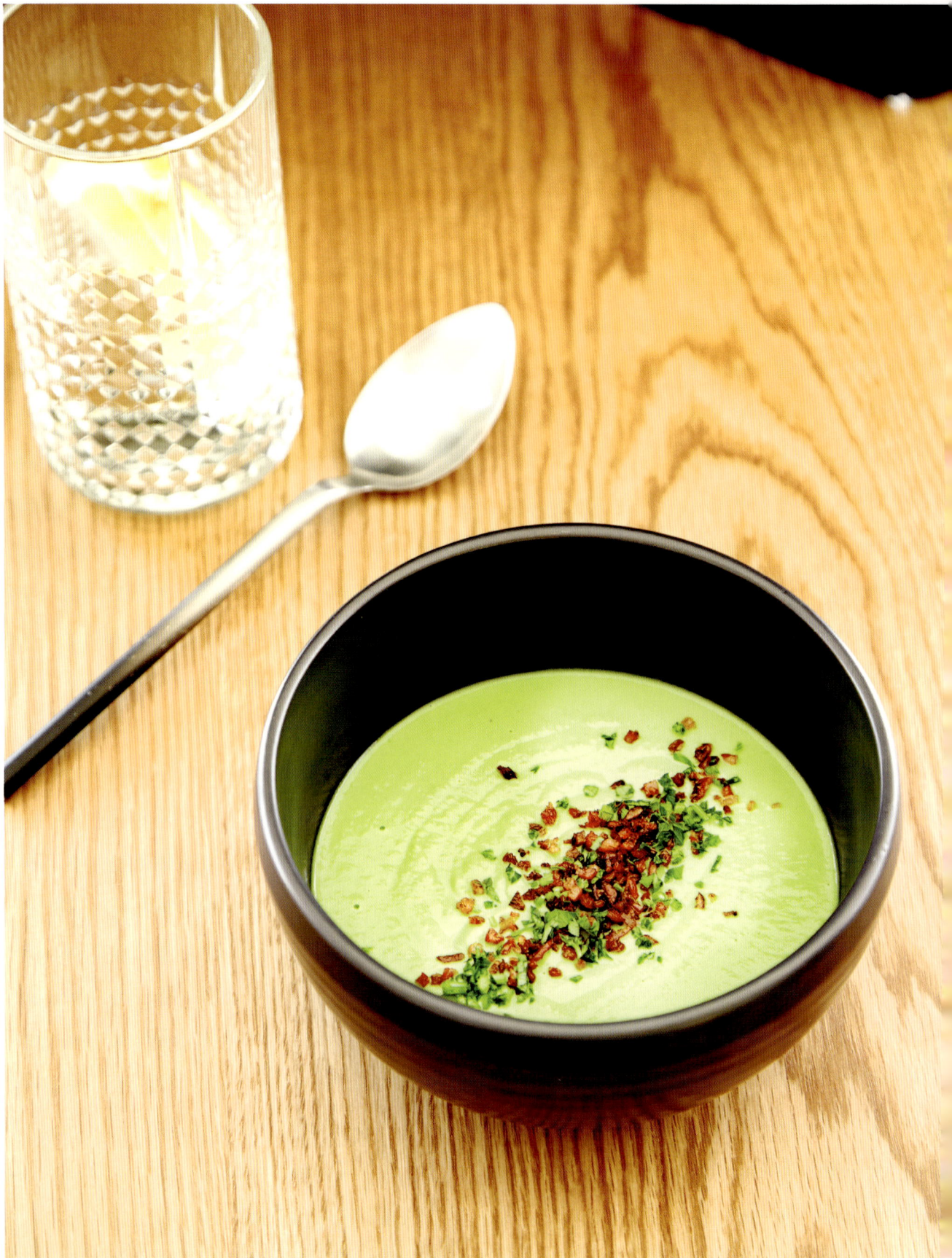

Packed with broccoli, spinach and peas the only thing that may be a little indulgent is the fried bread, which you can easy swap out for baked croutons.

BROCCOLI & PEA SOUP

Serves 4

Cooking Time: 1 hour 40 minutes

INGREDIENTS

- × 5 garlic cloves, unpeeled
- × 1 brown onion, roughly chopped
- × 1.5 litres (52 fl oz) chicken stock (see Basics, page 31 or unsalted if store bought)
- × 200 g (7 oz) broccoli, roughly chopped
- × 2 celery stalks, roughly chopped
- × 300 g (10½ oz) peas
- × 150 g (5½ oz) spinach
- × ¼ loaf sourdough bread
- × 1½ tablespoons olive oil, plus extra for drizzling
- × parmesan cheese, to serve
- × sea salt and cracked black pepper, to season

METHOD

Preheat the oven to 180˚C (350˚F/Gas 4). Grease a baking tray with a drizzle of olive oil.

Place the unpeeled garlic and onion on the baking tray. Place the tray in the oven and bake until garlic and onion are roasted (garlic will be soft when ready). Remove from the oven and leave to cool slightly. Peel the garlic.

Put the chicken stock in a large pot and place over medium heat. Add the broccoli, celery, peas and spinach to the pot. Add the onion and garlic. Bring the pot to a boil, then reduce the heat to a simmer and cover. Cook for 30 minutes with the lid on, then remove the lid and cook for a further 30 minutes. Season with sea salt and cracked black pepper, then remove from the heat and allow to cool for 10 minutes.

Meanwhile, remove the crusts from the bread, tear into bite-sized chunks and add to a mixing bowl. Drizzle with olive oil and toss to ensure the bread is coated, then season with a little sea salt.

Heat the olive oil in a large, non-stick frying pan over medium heat. When hot, add the bread, ensuring it is spread out evenly with no pieces on top of the other (do it in two batches if you pan is too small). Fry the bread until it is crunchy and brown on the bottom. When the bread is done on one side, turn each piece individually with a pair of tongs and cook again until browned. Remove from the pan and set aside in a bowl.

Using a blender, add the soup and purée in small batches until smooth.

When you are ready to serve the soup, heat it in a pot over low heat.

To serve, add soup to each bowl, top with the bread croutons, cracked black pepper and grated parmesan cheese.

From The Wise

Sardines may not be everyone's cup of tea but they are a pretty good fish for your pregnant partner to eat. High in protein, calcium and omega-3 fatty acids, these delicious little fishes are also low in mercury and metal content and a great source of vitamin B12 and vitamin D. For some reason a lot of people aren't fans of these delicacies so to tempt even the most anti-sardine types I have included a Greek style, mouth-watering recipe with a sauce of olive, tomatoes, lemon and my personal favourite fried bread (please feel free to make croutons in the oven or ditch the bread all together).

PAN FRIED SARDINE SALAD WITH TOMATOES, OLIVES & ROCKET

Serves 4
Cooking Time: 35 minutes

INGREDIENTS

- × 3 tablespoons olive oil, plus extra for frying
- × 4 tomatoes, diced
- × 1 red onion, thinly sliced
- × 2 garlic cloves, crushed
- × 50 g (13/4 oz) pitted black olives, roughly chopped
- × ¼ bunch flat-leaf (Italian) parsley, roughly chopped
- × 1 tablespoon white wine vinegar

- × ½ lemon, halved
- × ¼ loaf sourdough bread
- × 100 g (3½ oz) rocket (arugula)
- × 2 tablespoons plain (all-purpose) flour
- × 12 whole sardines, cleaned
- × sea salt and cracked black pepper, to season

METHOD

Heat 1 tablespoon of the olive oil in a frying pan over medium heat. When hot, add the tomatoes, onion, garlic, olives, parsley and white wine vinegar and stir. Squeeze one lemon quarter into the pan and cook until the tomatoes are soft and broken down. Remove from the heat and set aside.

Place the sourdough bread on a cutting board and carefully slice off the flat side crust.

Remove the bread inside until the sourdough is hollowed out, then tear the bread into bite-sized chunks and place in a large mixing bowl. Drizzle olive oil and a sprinkle of sea salt over the bread and toss well.

Continued ⤵

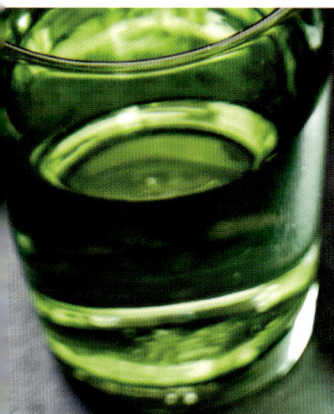

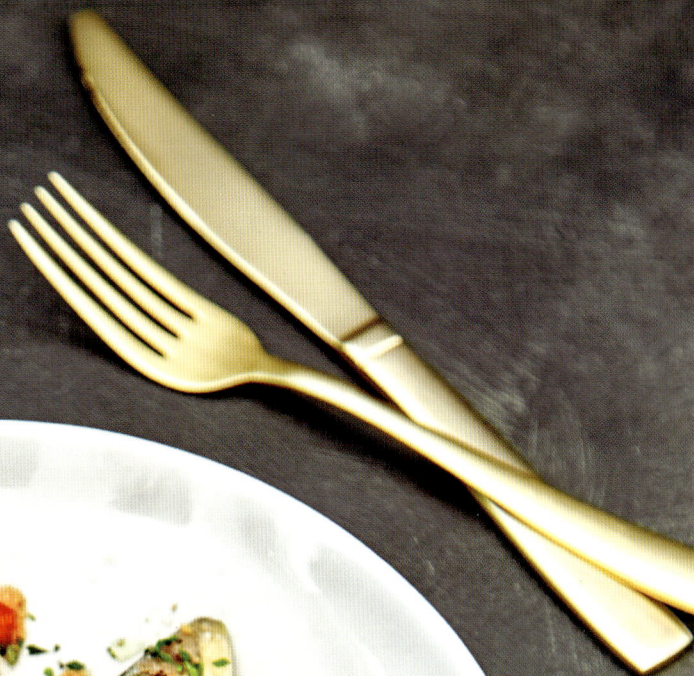

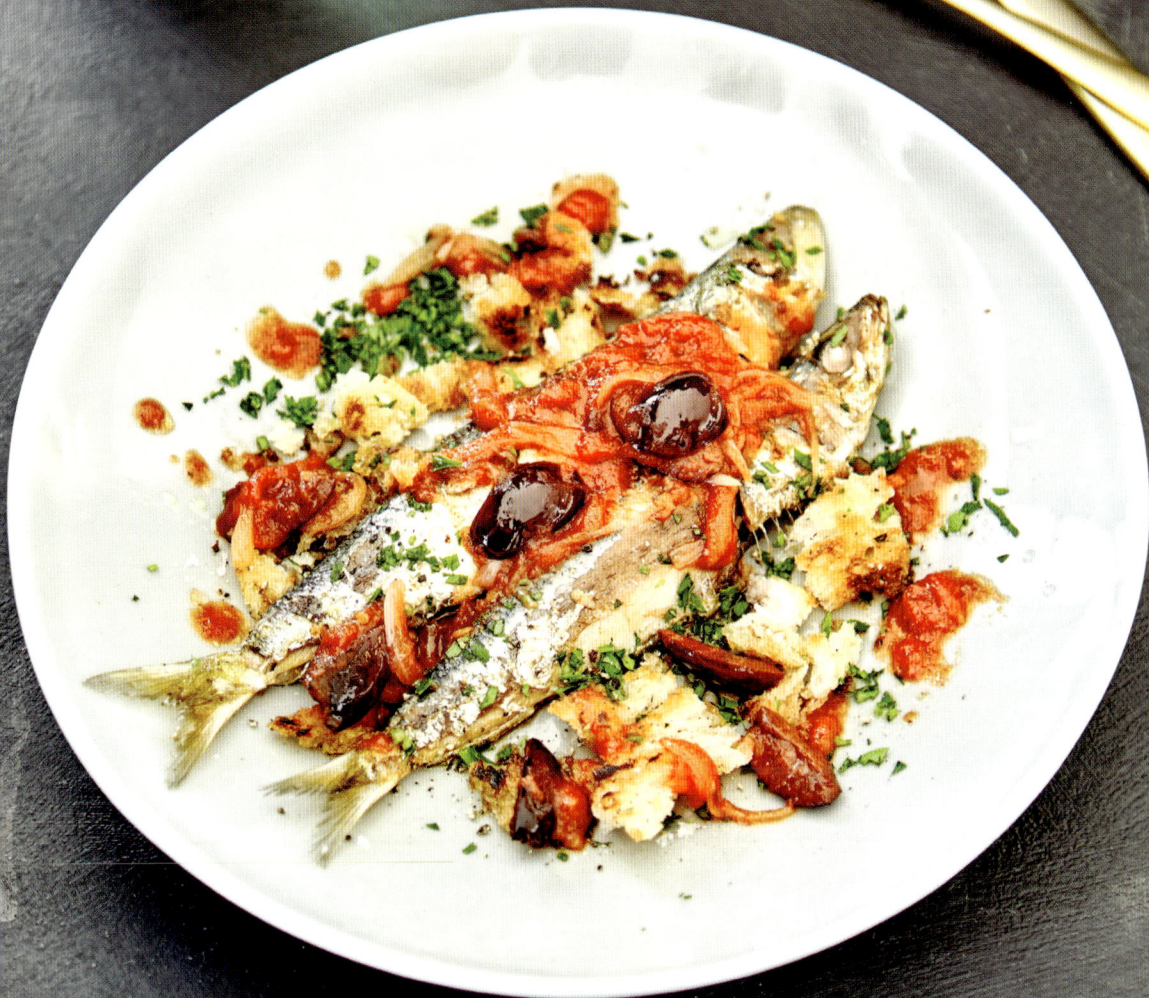

PAN FRIED SARDINE SALAD WITH TOMATOES, OLIVES & ROCKET CONTINUED...

Heat 1 tablespoon of the olive oil in a frying pan over medium heat. When hot, add the bread and cook on both sides until golden brown, then drain on paper towels.

Place the rocket in a bowl and drizzle with olive oil. Season with sea salt and some cracked black pepper.

Place the flour in a bowl and toss the sardines in the flour, ensuring they are coated.

Heat 1 tablespoon of the olive oil in a frying pan over medium heat. When hot, add the sardines and cook on both sides until golden.

To serve, place a little rocket on each plate, add three sardines, some bread and then spoon over the tomato mixture, finishing the dishes with a squeeze of the remaining lemon quarter.

SIMPLE SALADS

From The Wise

I know, I know. I can hear what you're saying. Salads are the easiest thing in the world make, any idiot can dump some lettuce in a bowl and top it with some oil. So, why should you pay all this money to read a recipe that you already know how to make?

Well there are several reasons, salads are healthy for both mother and baby, they are a great accompaniment for a myriad of different dishes and lastly, they are a reminder that we don't always have to make complex dishes for a dish to taste amazing.

ROCKET SALAD

Serves 4
Cooking Time: 5 minutes

INGREDIENTS
- × 120 g (41/4 oz) rocket (arugula)
- × 10 g (1/4 oz) parmesan cheese, grated
- × 2 tablespoons olive oil
- × sea salt and cracked black pepper, to season

METHOD
Place the rocket in a large mixing bowl and sprinkle with the parmesan cheese.
Drizzle with the olive oil and season with salt and pepper. Toss the salad well and serve immediately.

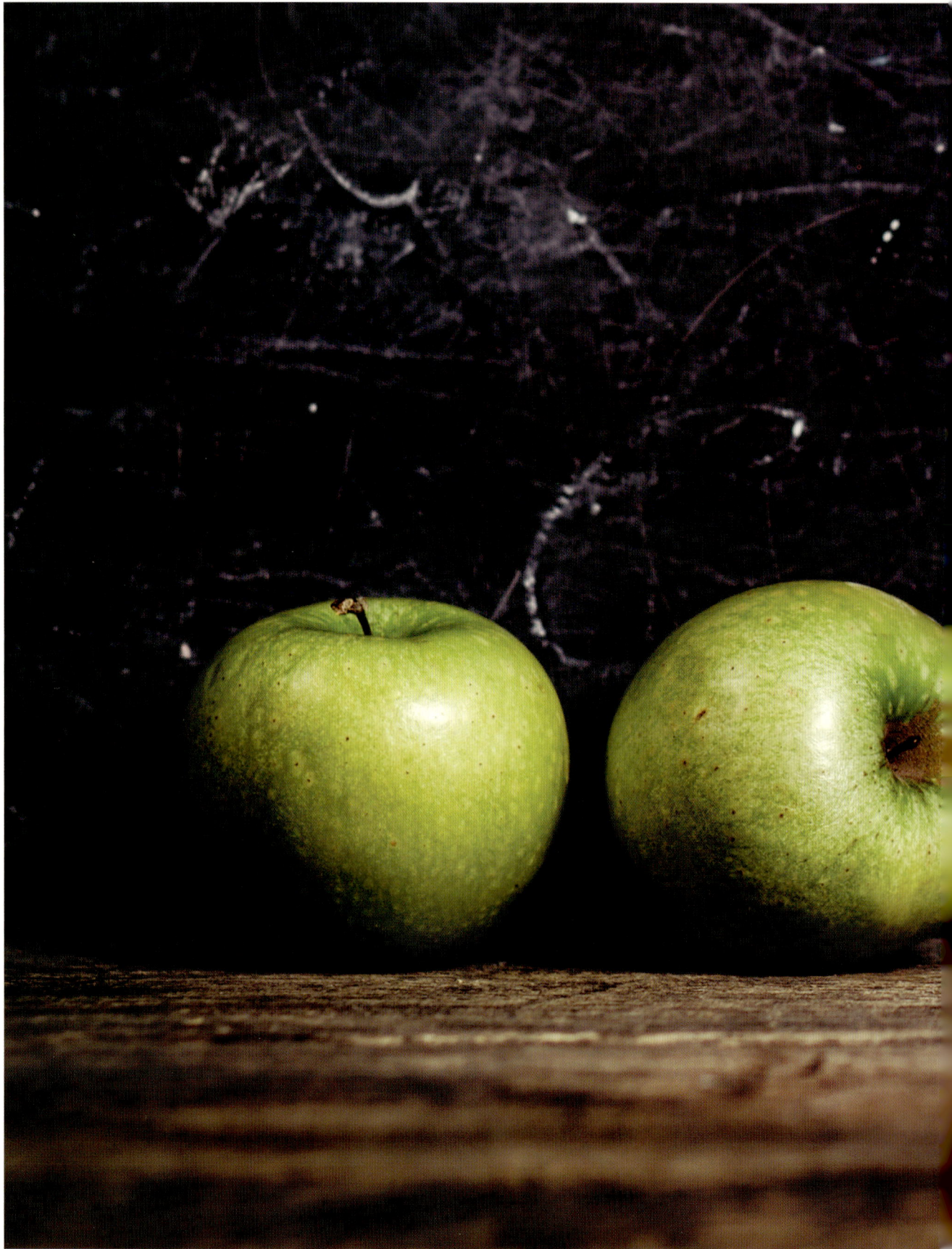

APPLE SALAD

Serves 4

INGREDIENTS

- × 1 tsp Dijon mustard
- × 2 tbsp apple cider vinegar
- × juice of ¼ of a lemon
- × 60 ml olive oil
- × 60 g (2 oz) white witlof leaves
- × 60 g (2 oz) red witlof leaves
- × 60 g (2 oz) green apple
- × sea salt
- × cracked black pepper

METHOD

Place Dijon mustard, apple cider vinegar and the juice of a quarter of a lemon into a mixing bowl and whisk together.

Drizzle in the olive oil and continue to whisk until an emulsion forms and the oil is combined. Set aside in an airtight container.

Pick the leaves off the red and white witlof and place them in a mixing bowl.

Shave the apple using a mandolin (watch the fingers!!!) or thinly slice with a knife and add to the mixing bowl.

Add a couple of tablespoons of the Dijon vinaigrette and season with sea salt and cracked black pepper.

Toss the salad well ensuring the vinaigrette coats all the leaves and the apple.

Serve.

SPINACH SALAD

INGREDIENTS

- ☓ 120 g (4 oz) baby spinach
- ☓ 2 tbsp good quality olive oil
- ☓ juice of ¼ of a lemon
- ☓ 1 tbsp balsamic vinegar
- ☓ sea salt
- ☓ cracked black pepper

METHOD

Wash and dry baby spinach.

Place the baby spinach into a large mixing bowl and squeeze over the lemon juice.

Drizzle the olive oil and balsamic vinegar over the top and season with salt and pepper.

Toss the salad well ensuring the oil and vinegar coats all the leaves.

Serve.

CRAVINGS

I think we can all agree that the eating fried chicken on a regular basis isn't a really good idea. So if you are going to do it, you'd better do it right. And when it comes to fried chicken, Japanese style karaage chicken right up there with the best of them. If you want to make unforgettable karaage chicken, the secret is getting the oil to just the right temperature. If the oil is too cool the chicken will soak it up and become greasy, while if it's too hot the outside will burn while the centre remains raw. So use a deep fryer or cooking thermometer to make sure that it's just right.

This dish comes with a warning: one taste of the crunchy fried goodness of the chicken with the zing of the pickled cabbage and the heat of the wasabi infused avocado, and you'll be hooked. So cook at your own peril, this dish is highly addictive!

KARAAGE CHICKEN ROLL WITH PICKLED VEGETABLES, WASABI & AVOCADO

Serves 2
Cooking Time: 45 minutes

INGREDIENTS

KARAAGE CHICKEN
- × 1 teaspoon dark sugar
- × 2 tablespoons light soy sauce
- × 1 small knob of ginger, grated
- × 1 garlic clove, crushed
- × 2 skinless chicken thighs, cut into chunks
- × 250 ml (9 fl oz) oil, for frying (I like peanut oil, but the choice is yours, just don't use olive oil)
- × 2 tablespoons potato flour

PICKLED CABBAGE, CUCUMBER & RADISH
- × 1½ teaspoons salt
- × 1 teaspoon sugar
- × 2 tablespoons rice wine vinegar
- × ¼ red cabbage, thinly sliced

- × ½ Lebanese (short) cucumber, thinly sliced
- × 2 radishes, thinly sliced

WASABI AVOCADO SPREAD
- × ½ ripe avocado, mashed
- × 2 coriander (cilantro) sprigs, finely chopped
- × ½ teaspoons wasabi (optional)
- × ¼ lime
- × 1 teaspoon sea salt
- × 1 teaspoon cracked black pepper

- × 2 fresh, crunchy absolutely amazing bakery bought white bread rolls
- × drizzle of Okonomi Sauce

(Continued)

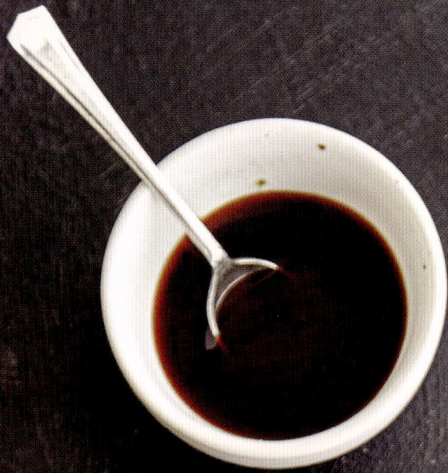

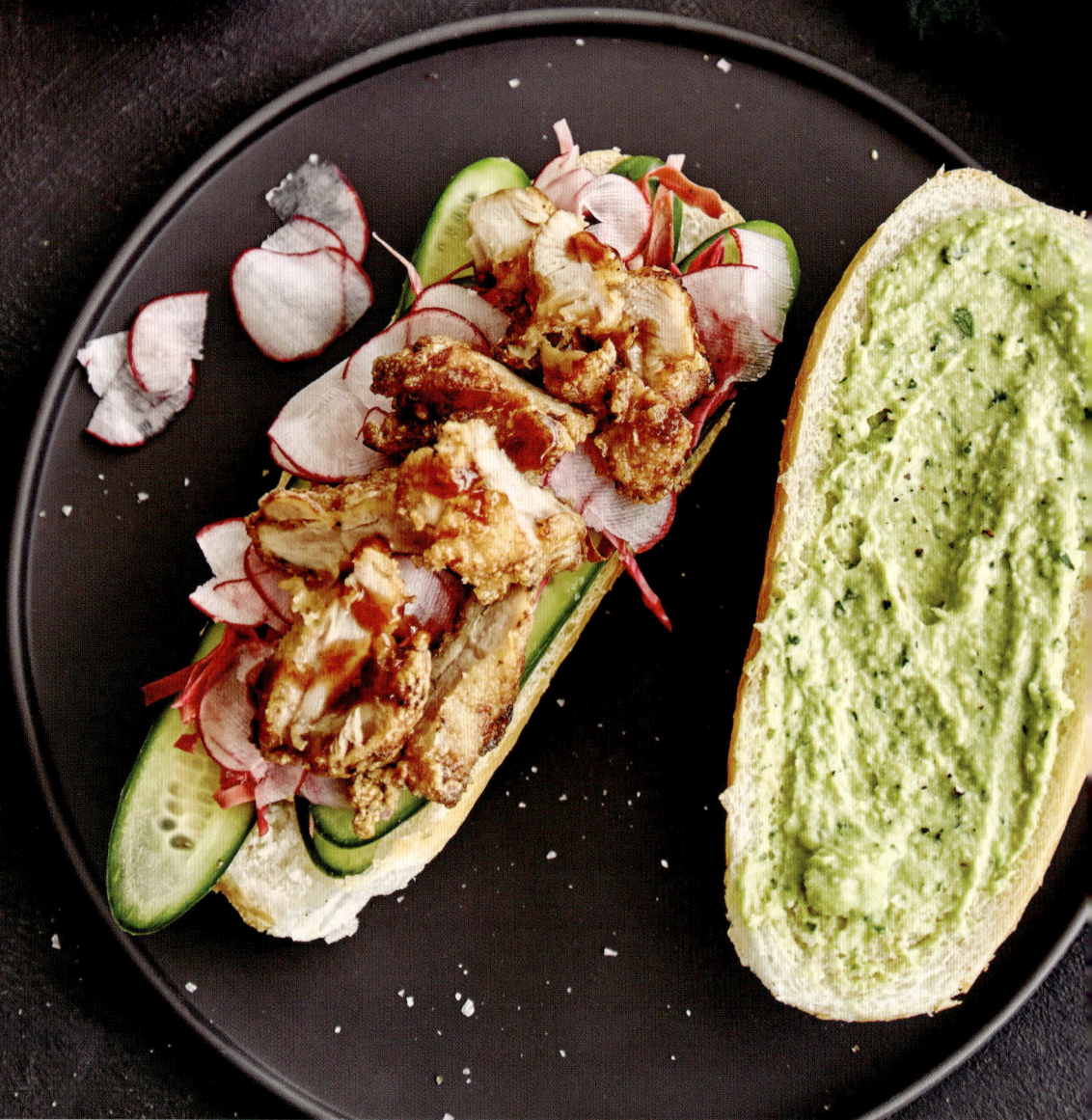

METHOD

To prepare the karaage chicken, place the dark sugar, light soy sauce, ginger and garlic into a mixing bowl and combine well. Add the chicken to the mixture, making sure the mixture coats the chicken well. Leave to marinate in the fridge for at least 30 minutes.

To make the pickled cabbage, cucumber and radish, place the salt, sugar and rice wine vinegar into a mixing bowl and combine well. Add the sliced cabbage, cucumber and radish. Leave to marinate for a minimum of 30 minutes.

To make the wasabi avocado spread, add the avocado, coriander and wasabi to a mixing bowl. Squeeze in the lime and season with sea salt and cracked black pepper. Mix well to combine. Refrigerate until needed.

Place the oil into a heavy-based saucepan or pot, ensuring it does not fill past halfway. Heat the oil to 180°C (350°F). You can also use a deep-fryer.

Remove the chicken from the marinade and place into a clean bowl. Add the potato flour, turning the chicken over with tongs and coating well. Shake off any excess flour and carefully add the chicken, one piece at time to the oil, frying until a browned and fully cooked through. (If you are in doubt slice one in half and check.)

Remove the chicken from the oil and place on a wire rack lined with paper towel and drain well.

Cut the bread rolls in half and coat one side liberally with the wasabi avocado spread. Squeeze any excess liquid from the pickled cabbage, cucumber and radish so they are moist but not soaking and place on top of the avocado. Add the chicken pieces and top with a drizzle of the Okonomi Sauce. Serve immediately.

Funtastic Baby Facts
Some newborns get acne.

This is a simple variant on the popular Thai fish cake and is easy to whip up as a snack. The chilli, lemongrass and ginger mix is also a great thing to keep in the fridge and use as a base for a quick noodle dish or stir fry.

PRAWN CAKES

Makes 10
Cooking Time: 30 minutes

INGREDIENTS

CHILLI, LEMONGRASS AND GINGER MIX
- × 7 red long chillies, deseeded and cut lengthways
- × 25 g (1 oz) ginger, julienned
- × 1 lemongrass stalk, chopped
- × 2 garlic cloves, thinly sliced
- × 1 shallot, thinly sliced
- × ½ lime, juiced
- × ½ teaspoons shrimp paste
- × 1 tablespoon fish sauce

- × 1 teaspoon dark sugar
- × 1/2 bunch coriander (cilantro), roughly chopped

- × 500 g (1 lb 2 oz) large green prawns (shrimp), peeled and deveined, roughly chopped
- × 125 g (4½ oz) plain (all-purpose) flour
- × 250 ml (9 fl oz) peanut oil (or any other type, just not olive)

Continued

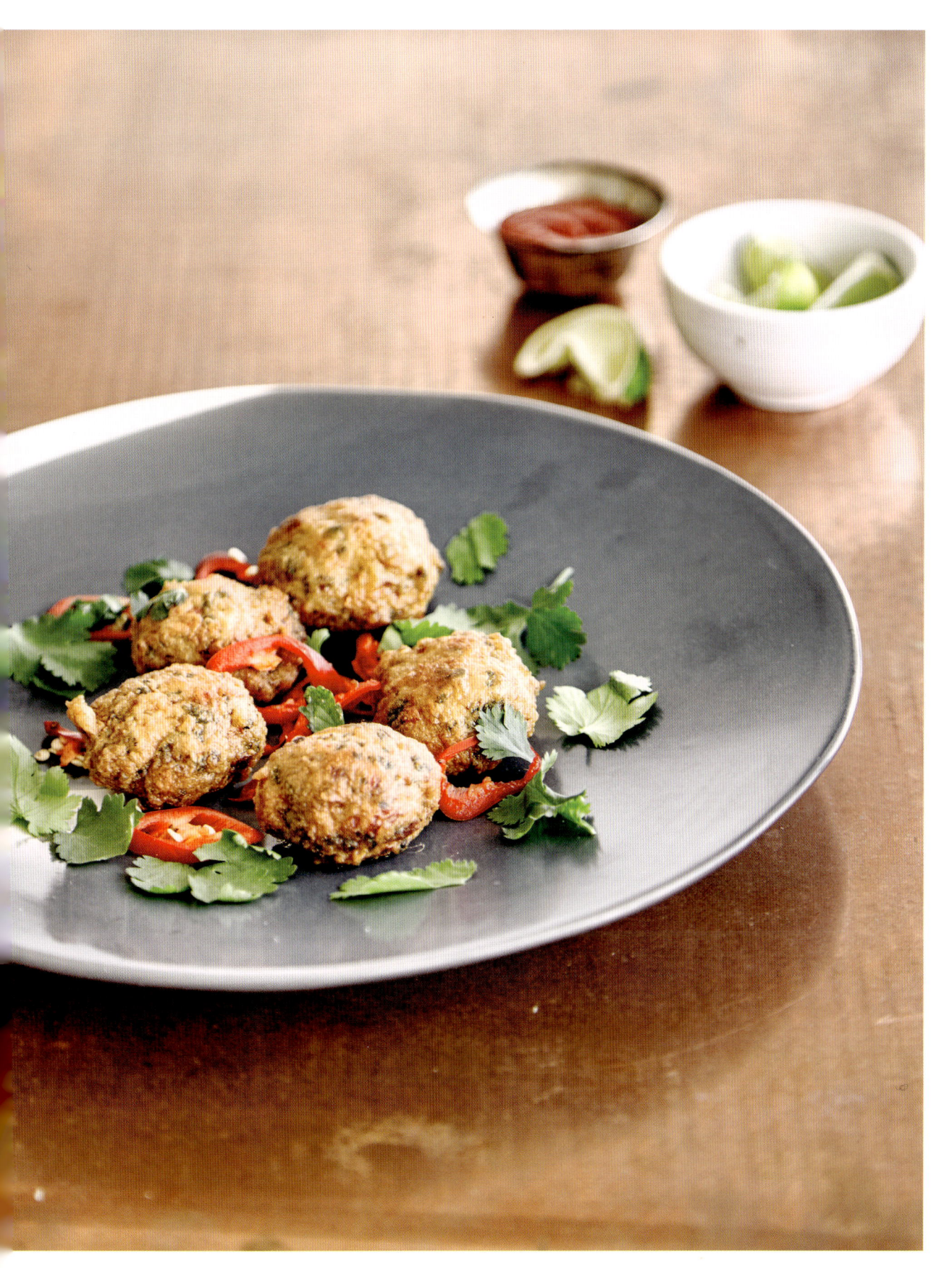

PRAWN CAKES CONTINUED...

To make the chilli, lemongrass and ginger mix, add all of the ingredients to a food processor. Cover with the lid and blend well, stopping to scrape down the sides so there are no chunks. Scrape out the mixture and place into an airtight container and store in the fridge (any leftover mixture is a great base for a noodle stir-fry or rice dish).

Add the prawns to the food processor with 2 heaped tablespoons of the chilli, lemongrass and ginger mix. Process a few times, but don't overdo it. (The mixture should still have chunks and texture, not a smooth prawn mousse). Scrape the prawn mixture into one bowl and the flour into another and lay a sheet of baking paper over a tray.

Grab a tablespoon-sized portion of the prawn mixture and form it into a rough ball between the palms of your hands. Press the ball gently between your palms to form a small cake.

Carefully place the prawn cake into the flour and coat well, then transfer to the baking paper lined tray. Repeat until all the mixture is used.

Place the oil in a heavy-based saucepan or pot ensuring it does not fill past halfway. Heat to 180°C (350°F). You can also use a deep-fryer.

Add the prawn cakes in small batches and cook until browned on one side, carefully turning and cooking on the other side. Place on paper towels to drain. Repeat until all the prawn mixture is used.

Serve as a snack with a sweet chilli or hot dipping sauce and a drizzle of fresh lime juice.

By no means am I suggesting that it is a good idea to made twenty pork belly bao for yourself and your partner to consume. That would be irresponsible. This is one of the dishes I cooked for my wife's baby shower. It's a great snack that you can hold with one hand, doesn't require anything more than a serving tray to put out for hungry guests and is downright delicious to eat. To make this dish you will need a steamer. For best results use a wok with a couple of large bamboo steamers stacked as you can fit in a lot of bread.

PORK BUN

Makes 20
Cooking Time: Overnight plus 2 hours and 55 minutes

INGREDIENTS

CRISPY PORK BELLY
- × 1 kg (2 lb 4 oz) pork belly (unscored)
- × handful of sea salt

BAO (CHINESE STEAMED BUN)
- × 3 tablespoons white sugar
- × 1 sachet instant yeast powder
- × 400 g (14 oz) plain (all-purpose) flour, plus extra for dusting

- × 1 teaspoon baking powder
- × ½ teaspoons salt
- × 1 tablespoon vegetable oil, plus extra for brushing the buns

- × 3 Lebanese (short) cucumbers, cut into long, thin strips
- × ½ bunch coriander (cilantro), roughly chopped
- × 100 ml (3⅓ fl oz) hoisin sauce

METHOD
The day before:

Place the pork belly skin side up on a chopping board and shave off any hairs with a disposable razor (when buying the pork belly ask for a piece that has not been scored). Boil some water. Place the pork belly into a large colander and carefully pour the boiling water onto the skin until it shrinks and retracts. Remove the pork belly from the sink and place it back on the chopping board.

Using a carving fork, regular fork or in a pinch, a metal skewer, poke hundreds of holes into the skin, making sure you get a good coverage across the entire surface (this will take a while and is quiet a laborious and boring task).

Grab a handful of sea salt and sprinkle over the top of the skin, then cover and put in the pork belly in the fridge overnight (if you forget to do this part the night before make sure you do it first thing in the morning and keep it in the fridge for 3–4 hours).

(Continued)

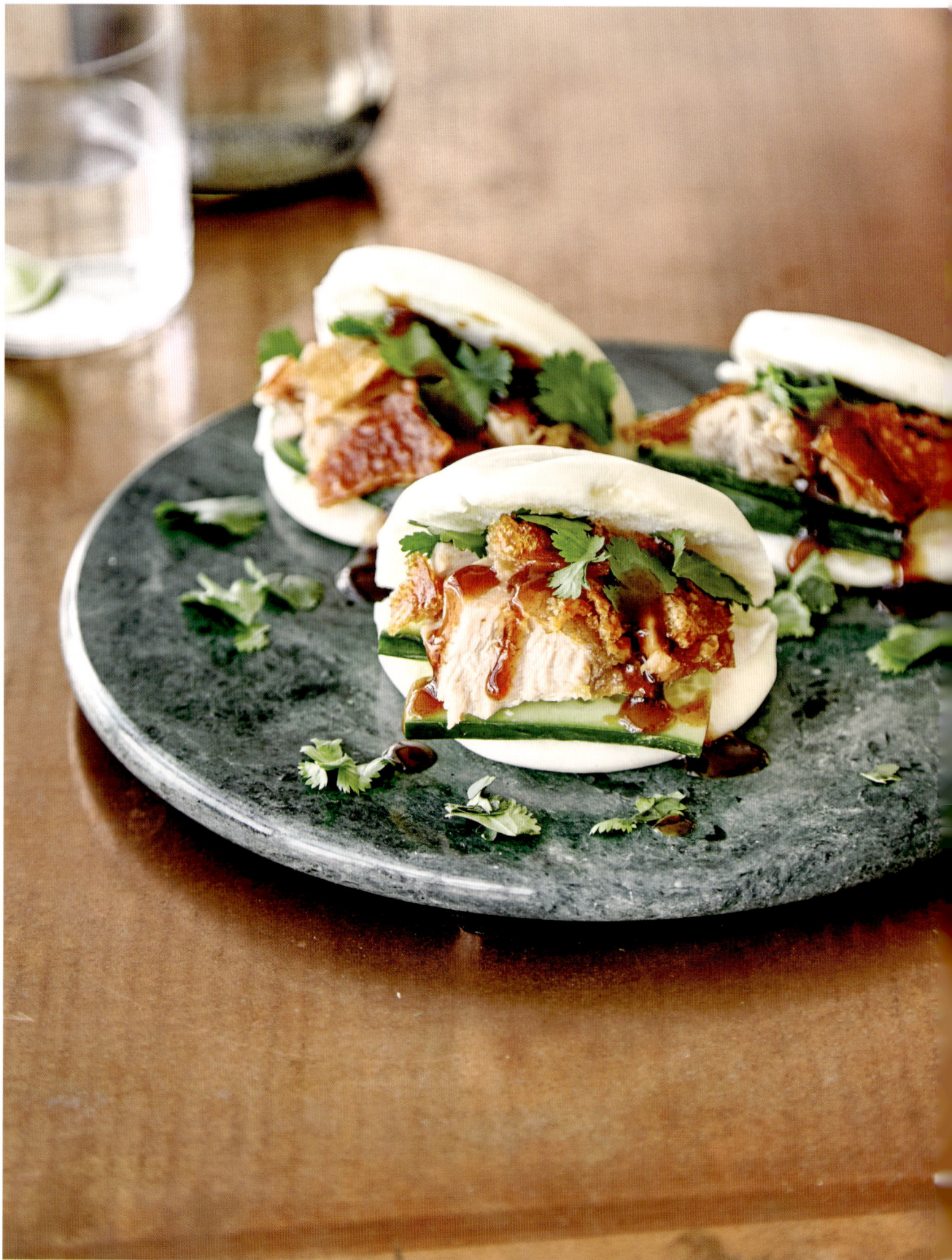

PORK BUN CONTINUED...

To make the steamed buns, pour the sugar and 250 ml (9 fl oz) of warm water in a mixing bowl and add the yeast, stirring to combine. Cover the bowl with a tea towel and set aside for 10 minutes. The mixture should bubble or foam on the top (if it doesn't it means the yeast has not activated, so you'll have to discard it and start again). Add 1 tablespoon of vegetable oil to the yeast mixture.

Sift the flour and baking powder into a large mixing bowl or a stand mixer, then add the salt. If you are making the bread by hand, stir the dry ingredients with a wooden spoon, then slowly drizzle in the yeast mixture, stirring until all of the liquid is combined and a rough dough is formed.

If you are using a stand mixer, attach the paddle and combine for 1 minute, then stop and attach the dough hook and slowly drizzle in the yeast mixture until all of the liquid is combined and a rough dough is formed.

If you are making the bread by hand, turn the dough out onto a floured work surface and knead for 10 minutes (the dough should be shiny and elastic but not sticky). If you are using a stand mixer, knead the dough for 3–4 minutes.

Form the dough into a ball then place it in a mixing bowl, cover with a tea towel and leave to stand for 2 hours.

Preheat the oven to 220°C (425°F).

About 30 minutes after making the dough, remove the pork from the fridge and place skin side down on a wire rack in a roasting tray. Place the pork belly in the oven and roast for 25–30 minutes, depending on the thickness of the meat. Remove the tray from the oven and carefully flip the meat over. Cook skin side up for 30 minutes. Remove from the oven.

Preheat the oven grill (broiler) to high. When the grill is very hot, place the roasting tray underneath and cook for 5–10 minutes, or until the skin is crispy and blistered. Rest for 15 minutes.

The bread dough should have doubled in size by now. Punch the dough down and place it on a floured work surface. Using a knife, divide the dough into 20 portions forming each portion into a ball and setting aside underneath a tea towel.

Pour a little vegetable oil into a bowl and grab a pastry brush. Using one portion at a time, grab the dough and place on the floured surface. Using a rolling pin, gently roll it out into and elongated oval shape (stretch it with your hands if you are not happy with how they look.)

Lightly brush the surface of the dough with the vegetable oil and fold it over so the ends meet, then carefully return it under the tea towel and repeat with the rest of the dough.

Half-fill your wok or steamer with water and place over medium heat.

Place your bamboo steamer or steamer basket on the workbench and tear off a piece of baking paper that is roughly the same size as the width of the entire steamer. Fold the baking paper in half and then fold the top corners over to the bottom centre of the paper to make two triangles. Fold the two triangles together to make one (should look like a pointed paper plane with no wings). Hold the pointed tip of the folded baking paper above centre of the steamer and measure to the edge marking with your finger and cutting off any excess in

PORK BUN CONTINUED...

an arc shape. Snip the tip from the centre and unfold, should be a steamer sized circle of paper with a hole in the middle. Lay the cartouche on the bottom of the bamboo steamer or steamer basket and gently place the buns inside spacing so they have room (do this step in batches if you can't fit them in).

When the water is boiling place the bamboo steamer or steamer basket over the top and cook for 5 minutes. Remove the bao from the steamer and repeat until all the dough is cooked.

Slice the pork belly into strips. Open the bao and smear a teaspoon of the hoisin sauce.

Fold the cucumber strips, stack with lots of crispy pork belly and finish with some coriander leaves.

MY DAUGHTER CALLS ME MUMMY

There is nothing quite like the greeting you receive from your little one when you open the front door and walk into your home. Their entire face lights up, eyes filled with a love that only a child can have for their parents as they run towards you with arms open wide happily calling out, 'Mummy, Mummy, Mummy'.

That is of course, unless you're Daddy.

Now, my little girl can say quite a few words and phrases, she has mastered the alibility to say 'yes' and 'no', is happy to tell me what is 'yucky' or 'yummy', she recites the names of her favourite cartoon characters and with a little prompting she can even imitate the sounds of several animals.

For some reason however the word Daddy still eludes her.

I was thrilled when my daughter was able to say 'Mummy', the obvious joy it brought my wife was more than enough to keep me happily waiting in expectation for that magical day when she proudly proclaimed 'Daddy' for the first time. But as the weeks passed and her vocabulary increased, she was soon able to name several animals we passed on the street, to count to three and sing along to her favourite songs, but no amount of cajoling could coax that word from her lips and I started to wonder why I was not being acknowledged by her at all.

This feeling continued until one night when we were sitting on the couch filling the moments between her nightly bottle and bedtime she pointed at me with a big smile on her face and said 'Mummy'. I suddenly realised that she had in fact been acknowledging me all along and I was Mummy as well.

Some men may find this a little emasculating but to tell you the truth I think it's pretty cute and I wear my Mummy badge with honour. And although it wouldn't hurt her to learn how to say Daddy just once, I take solace in those magical moments when her face lights up and she runs towards me, her Mummy, for a big hug. Because as friends who have teenagers have told me, enjoy it now, it doesn't last forever.

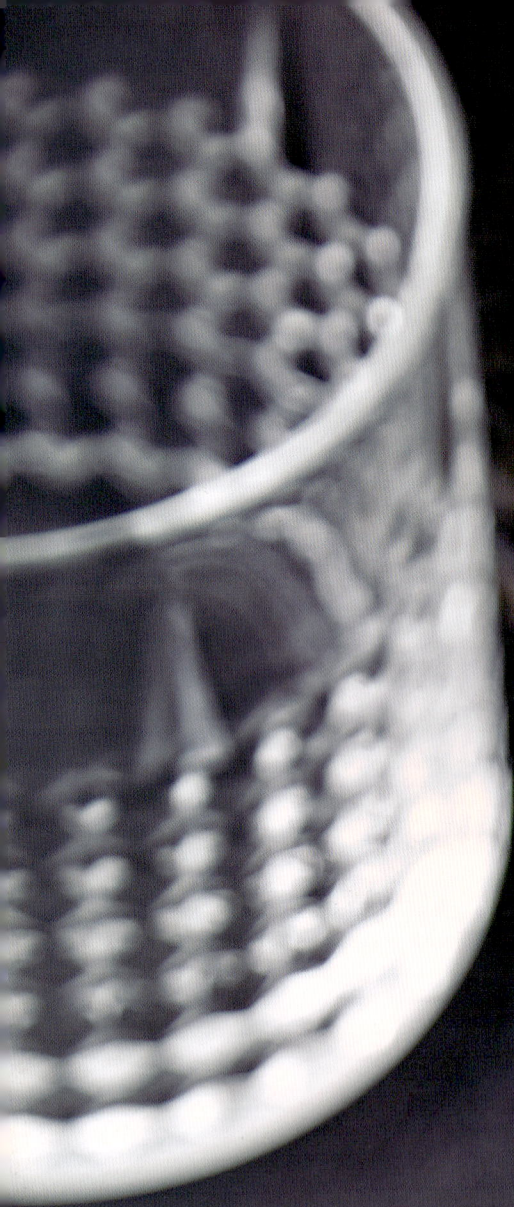

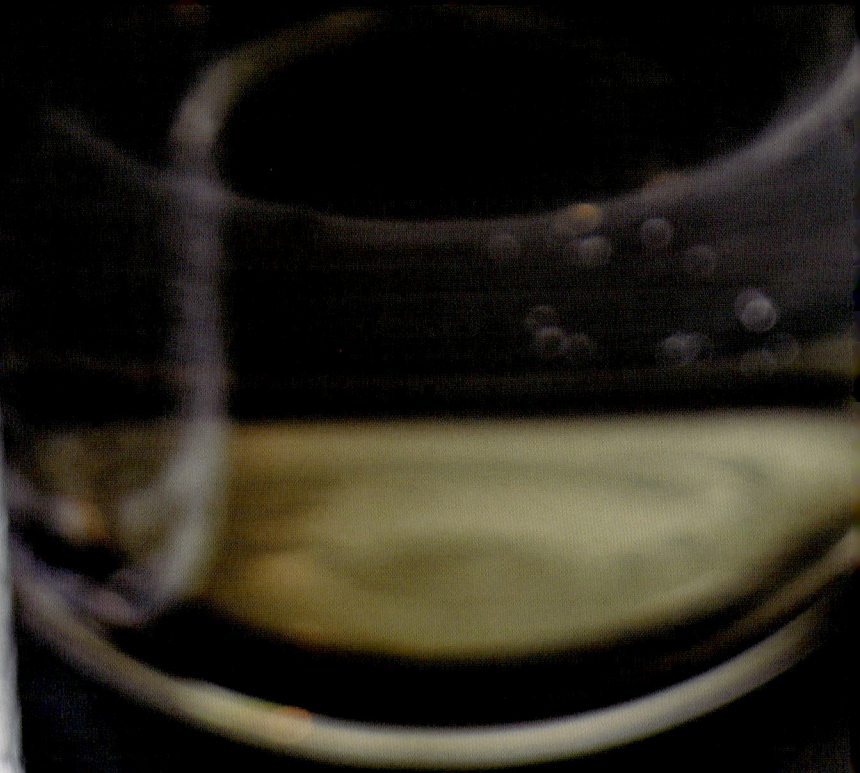

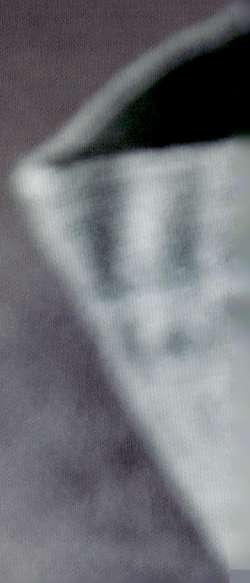

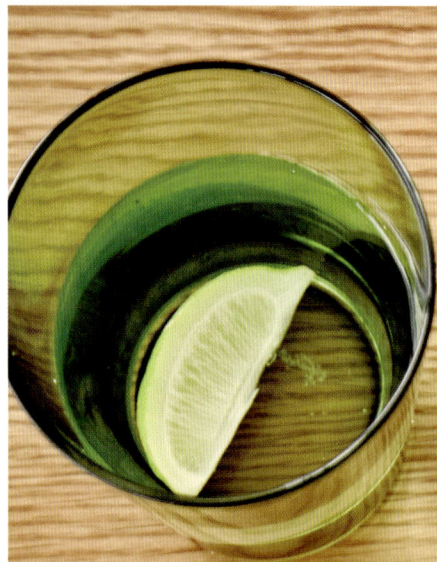

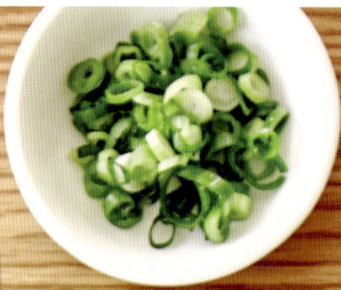

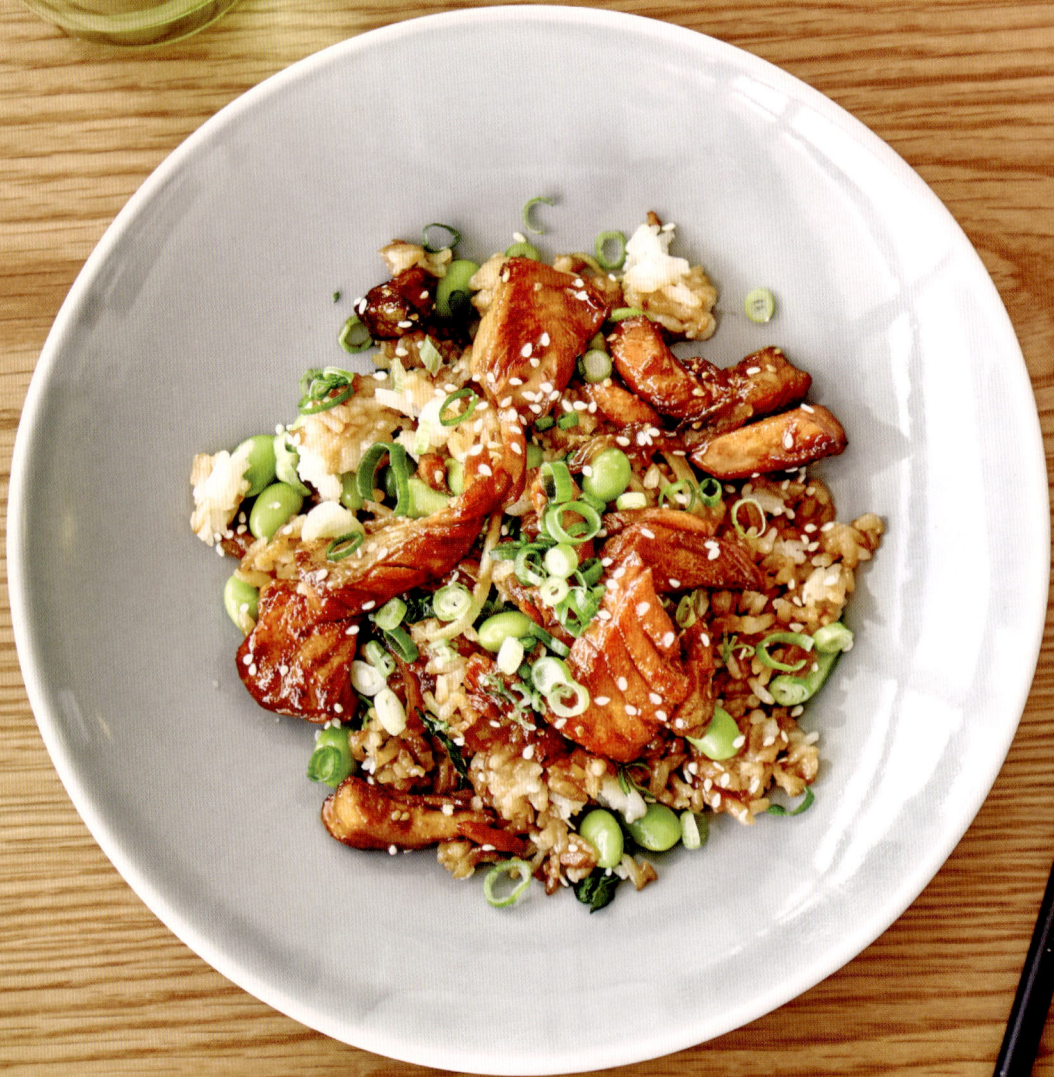

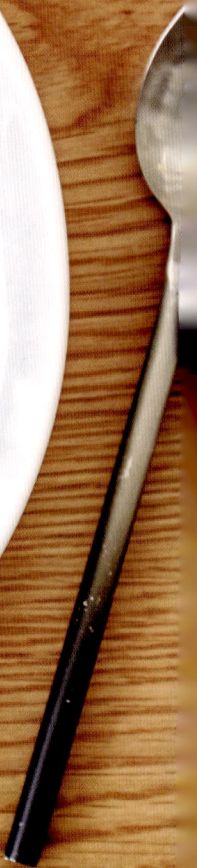

Salmon is a great fish to serve while your partner is pregnant (remember to limit it to 2—3 serves a week), because it's high in protein, omega-3 fatty acids and vitamin D while relatively low in mercury content. The only downside is that the fish has to be served cooked through so a delectable medium salmon steak or salmon sashimi are off the menu. This dish however is a good compromise, cooking the salmon through while not becoming dry or bland.

TERIYAKI SALMON RICE BOWL

Serves 4
Preparation & Cooking Time: 50 minutes

INGREDIENTS

- × 3 tablespoons dark soy sauce
- × 2 teaspoons brown sugar
- × 2 garlic cloves, crushed
- × 25 g (1 oz) ginger
- × 2 salmon fillets, cut into 1.5 cm (½ in) thick pieces
- × 200 g (7 oz) Japanese short grain rice
- × 2 tablespoons rice vinegar

- × 150 g (5½ oz) edamame
- × 1 tablespoon vegetable oil
- × 2 bunches of baby bok choy (pak choy), roughly chopped
- × 1 spring onion (scallion) stalk, thinly sliced
- × sesame seed, to garnish

METHOD

Add the dark soy sauce, brown sugar, garlic to a mixing bowl. Slice off a piece of the ginger (about a third), and grate into bowl mixing the ingredients well. Peel the remaining ginger, julienne and set aside for garnish.

Add the salmon pieces, coat and set aside in the fridge for 30 minutes to marinate.

Put the rice into a rice cooker cover with 200 ml (7 fl oz) water and cook as per instructions until done OR place rice in a saucepan, cover with 400 ml (14 fl oz) water and bring to boil. Drop heat to a simmer and cook until the water is absorbed and rice is tender yet firm which will take 10-15 minutes. Leave to stand in steam for a further 10 minutes, then add rice vinegar and fluff the rice.

Place a steamer over medium heat and bring the water to a simmer. Add the edamame to the steamer and steam for 5 minutes.

Heat the vegetable oil in a non-stick frying pan over medium heat. When the pan is hot, add the salmon and cook until caramelised on both sides. Add the bok choy and edamame and toss in the pan for 30 seconds. Remove from the heat.

To serve, add some rice to a bowl then top with the teriyaki salmon, bok choy, edamame and garnish with spring onions, ginger and a pinch of sesame seeds.

When it comes to making tacos there is nothing better than making your own tortillas but this can be a very time-consuming thing to do so nobody is going to blame you if you use store-bought ones. If you are running short of time you could also skip making the salsa and just make the guacamole, topping the fish off with some coriander, thinly sliced red onion and a splash of hot sauce.

FISH TACO WITH A ROASTED CORN & BLACK BEAN SALSA

Serves 4
Cooking Time: 1 hour 10 minutes

INGREDIENTS

FLOUR TORTILLAS
× 160 g (5¾ oz) plain (all-purpose) flour, plus extra for dusting
× ½ teaspoons table salt
× 3 tablespoons sunflower oil
× 100 ml (3½ fl oz) warm water

ROASTED CORN AND BLACK BEAN SALSA
× 1 ear of corn
× ½ teaspoon chipotle powder or smoked paprika
× ¼ red onion, finely diced
× 2 coriander (cilantro) sprigs, finely chopped
× 1 tablespoon apple cider vinegar
× 1 teaspoon molasses
× 1 tablespoon sunflower oil
× 65 g (2½ oz) black beans
× sea salt, to season

GUACAMOLE
× 1 avocado, diced
× 1 tomato, quartered, seeds discarded, diced
× 1 garlic clove, crushed
× ¼ bunch coriander (cilantro), roughly chopped
× pinch of cumin
× pinch of chipotle powder or smoked paprika
× juice of ½ a lime
× splash of hot sauce (optional)
× sea salt and cracked black pepper, to season

× 2 snapper or kingfish fillets
× sea salt and cracked black pepper, to season
× juice of 1/2 a lime
× 1 tablespoon sunflower oil
× ¼ bunch coriander (cilantro), roughly chopped
× ¼ red onion, thinly sliced
× splash of hot sauce (optional)

Preheat the oven to 180˚C (350˚F/Gas 4). Lightly grease a baking tray with sunflower oil.

To make the tortillas, place the flour and salt into a food processor or a stand mixer (a low setting to start with) and mix together. Add the sunflower oil and combine. Continue to mix the flour, carefully pouring the warm water into the bowl in a thin stream, watching as it clumps until a rough dough is formed. If you are using a food processor, turn out the dough onto a lightly floured work surface and knead for 8 minutes, or knead in the stand mixer for 5 minutes. Cover dough in plastic wrap and set aside in the fridge for 30 minutes.

To make the roasted corn and black bean salsa, place the corn on the baking tray. Drizzle some sunflower oil over the corn and sprinkle the chipotle powder or smoked paprika, ensuring you have coated all sides. Roast in the oven until cooked and the outside is slightly blackened. Remove the corn from the oven and leave to cool slightly.

When cool enough to handle, hold the cob vertically on the chopping board, running a knife down each side and slicing off all of the kernels.

Add the corn, red onion and coriander to a mixing bowl and mix well to combine. Add the apple cider vinegar, molasses, sunflower oil and beans and toss together well. Season with sea salt and set aside.

To make the guacamole, add the avocado to a mixing bowl and mash into a paste with a fork (you could also run it through a potato ricer if you prefer a smoother finish) Add the tomato, garlic and coriander and mix together. Add the cumin, chipotle powder or smoked paprika, juice of half a lime and hot sauce (optional) and combine. Taste and season with sea salt and cracked black pepper then set aside in the refrigerator.

Remove the tortilla dough from the fridge and divide into eight portions. Flour the workbench and press each piece of dough into a roundish disc.

Grab a rolling pin and roll out the dough into desired shape, placing the pin across one side and quarter turning after several rolls. Place each finished piece beneath a sheet of baking paper and continue until all the dough is rolled out.

Heat a dry cast iron skillet over medium heat until hot (If you don't have a cast iron skillet you can use a normal frying pan) and add the dough. Flip the tortilla when it is mottled and slightly blackened and cook on the other side. When done, remove from the pan and wrap in foil to keep warm. Repeat this process with the remaining dough.

Place the fish onto a plate and squeeze the juice of half a lime over the top, then season with sea salt and cracked black pepper.

Heat the sunflower oil in a frying pan over medium heat. When hot, place the fish in the pan and cook until brown on one side, then using a spatula carefully flip over and continue until the fish is cooked through (Break a piece apart to check). Remove the fish from the pan and break into chunks.

Remove the tortillas from the foil and place one piece of bread on each plate. Spoon on a generous amount of guacamole onto the tortilla and spread. Add the fish, hot sauce (optional) and several spoonsful of the roasted corn and black bean salsa. Top the taco with a few slices of the red onion, coriander and serve.

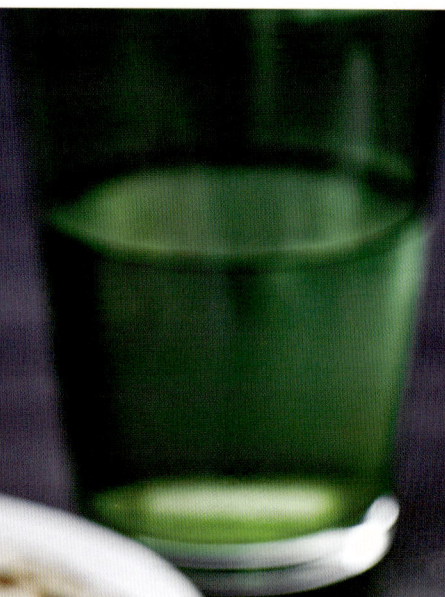
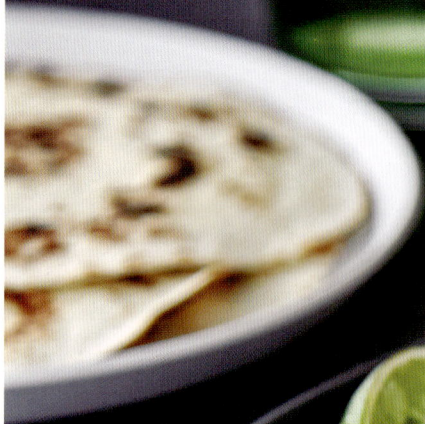
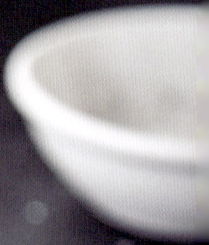
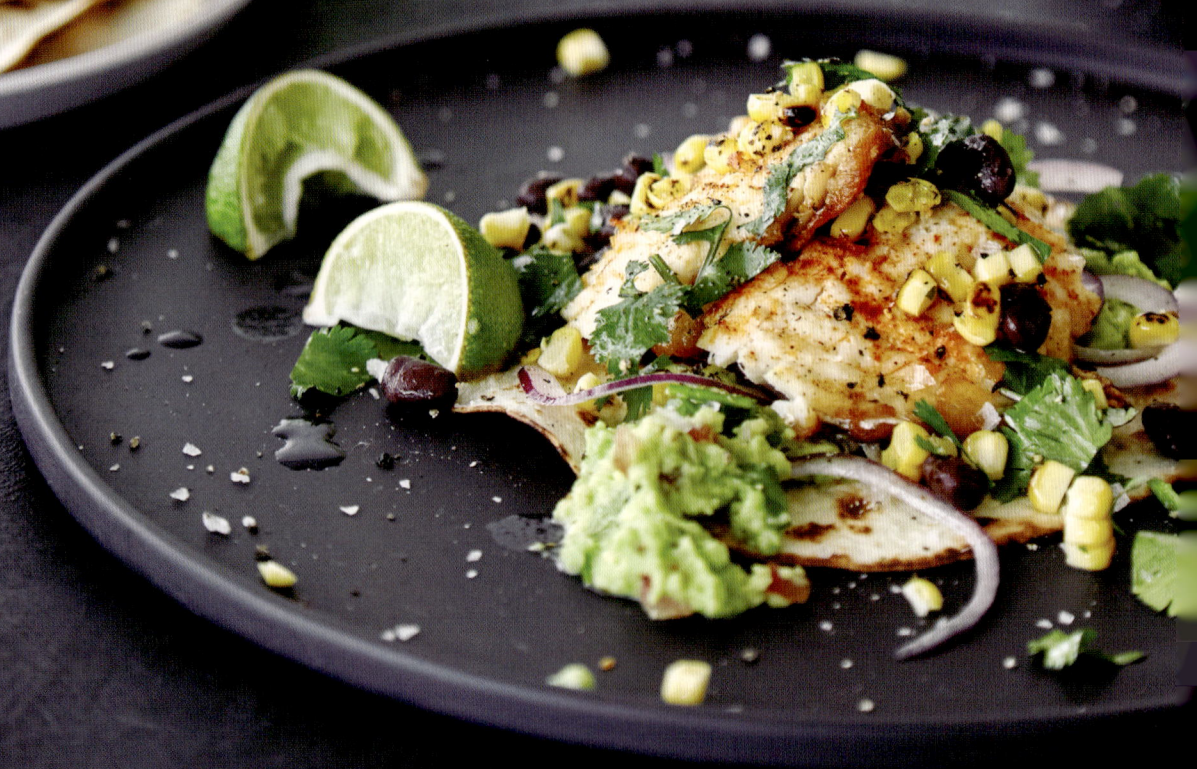

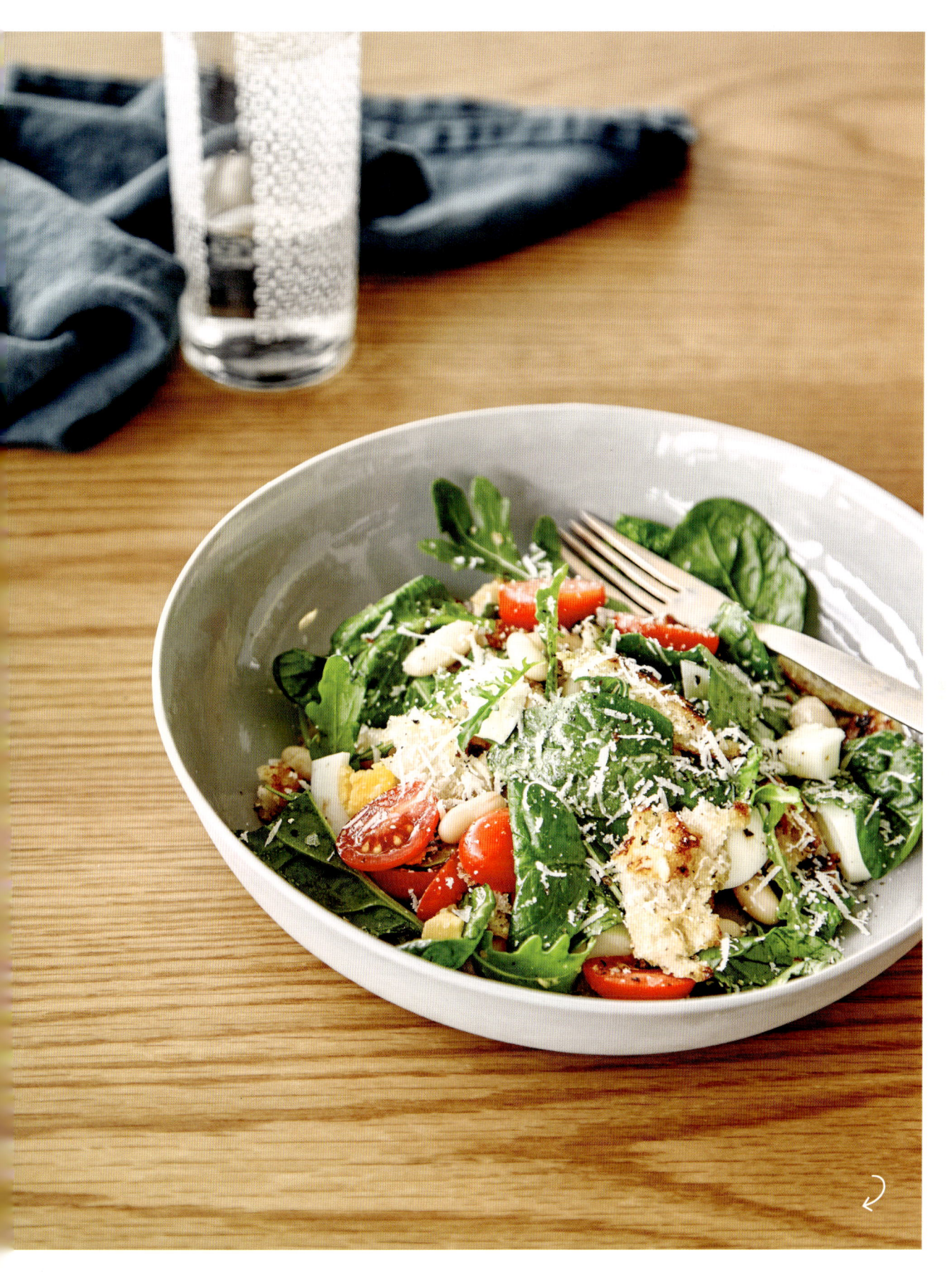

This is a pregnancy-friendly version of a classic dish called Panzanella, a Tuscan salad of bread and tomatoes. This was a favorite in our house while my wife was pregnant and I have fortified the recipe a bit with a few pregnancy friendly ingredients and added fried bread for a bit of a treat (if you prefer the healthier option feel free to toast the bread in the oven to make croutons).

TOMATO & CANNELLINI BEAN SALAD WITH ROCKET, SPINACH & FRIED SOURDOUGH BREAD

Serves 4
Cooking Time: 35 minutes

INGREDIENTS

- × 3 eggs
- × ½ loaf sourdough bread
- × 4 tablespoons olive oil, plus extra for salad dressing
- × 120 g (4¼ oz) baby English spinach
- × 120 g (4¼ oz) rocket (arugula)

- × 175 g (6 oz) cherry tomatoes, halved
- × sea salt and cracked black pepper, to season
- × ¼ bunch basil, leaves roughly torn
- × 400 g (14 oz) cannellini beans, drained
- × 20 g (¾ oz) parmesan cheese

METHOD

Bring a saucepan of water to a rolling boil and add the eggs. Cook until hard-boiled, then remove from the water and set aside. (How long it takes to hard boil an egg really depends on the size and can range from between 10–15 minutes. If you are unsure, cook it for longer.)

While the eggs are cooking, place the sourdough bread on a cutting board and carefully slice off the flat side crust. Remove the bread inside until the sourdough is hollowed out, then tear the bread into bite-sized chunks and place into a large mixing bowl.

Drizzle 2 tablespoons of the olive oil over the bread and some sea salt, tossing well.

Heat the remaining olive oil in a large, non-stick frying pan over medium heat. When hot, add the bread, ensuring it is spread out evenly with no pieces on top of the other (do it in 2 batches if you pan is too small). Fry the bread until it is crunchy and brown on the bottom (resist the temptation to move the bread, just check one piece with some tongs.)

When the bread is done on one side, turn each piece individually with a pair of tongs and cook again until browned. Remove from the pan and set aside.

Place the baby English spinach and rocket in a large mixing bowl. Season the tomatoes liberally with salt and pepper and add to the bowl. Add the basil leaves. Peel the eggs and roughly chop, then add to the bowl along with the bread and the beans. Grate the parmesan over the top and drizzle the olive oil over, tossing the salad well.

Funtastic Baby Facts
Newborns have more tastebuds than adults.

This dish is a quick and easy version of a hamburger with a lamb & chickpea patty topped with hummus and tabouli that packs a serious nutritional punch without skimping out on the flavour. If you are in a bit of a rush, feel free to ditch making the tabouli (although it is my favourite part of the dish) and if you feel like adding a bit of extra flavour you could always top the burger with a couple of slices of pan fried haloumi cheese!

LAMB & CHICKPEA BURGER WITH TABOULI

Serves 4
Cooking Time: 1 hour

INGREDIENTS

LAMB & CHICKPEA PATTY
- × 200 g (7 oz) tinned chickpeas, drained
- × 2 oregano sprigs, leaves finely chopped
- × 80 g (23/4 oz) pine nuts
- × 1 tablespoon cumin
- × 1 tablespoon sesame seeds
- × ½ teaspoons red chilli powder
- × 1 teaspoon nutmeg
- × 300 g (10½ oz) lean minced (ground) lamb
- × 1 teaspoon salt
- × 1 tablespoon cracked black pepper

TABOULI
- × 70 g (2 ½ oz) burghul (bulgur)
- × 2 tomatoes, seeds discarded, diced
- × juice of ⅔ of a lemon

- × 2 spring onions (scallions), thinly sliced
- × 1 bunch flat-leaf (Italian) parsley, roughly chopped
- × ¼ bunch mint, roughly chopped
- × 3 tablespoons olive oil
- × sea salt and cracked black pepper, to season

- × 80 g (23/4 oz) baby English spinach
- × 2 tablespoons olive oil
- × 1 loaf Turkish bread
- × 4 tablespoons hummus (see Basics, page 36 or store bought.)
- × 2 Lebanese (short) cucumbers, thinly sliced lengthways
- × 2 tomatoes, sliced
- × ½ red onion, thinly sliced
- × chilli sauce (optional)

METHOD

To make the lamb patties, place a small, dry frying pan over medium heat, add the pine nuts and and cook until toasted. Set aside in a bowl.

Return the same pan to the heat and dry roast the cumin, sesame seeds, red chilli powder and nutmeg until fragrant and add to the bowl.

Place the chickpeas, oregano and the bowl of nuts and spices into a food processor and pulse the mixture a few times until you have a chunky mash.

Add the lamb to the food processor, season well with salt and pepper, then pulse the mixture until everything is combined. Scrape the mixture out into a bowl and cover, placing it in the fridge for 15 minutes.

To make the tabouli, add the burghul, diced tomato and the juice of half a lemon to a mixing bowl and cover with a tea towel and leave to stand for 30 minutes.

Preheat the oven to 180˚C (350˚F/Gas 4). Place the baby English spinach into a bowl and add the olive oil tossing together well. Remove the lamb mixture from the fridge and form into four patties.

Heat the olive oil in a large cast iron skillet or oven-proof frying pan over medium heat until it is very hot. Place the lamb patties in the pan and fry for 3 minutes on each side. Place the pan in the oven and cook for a further 4 minutes. Remove the pan from the oven and place the lamb patties on a cutting board to rest.

Add 3 tablespoons of olive oil to the tabouli and season with salt and pepper.

Cut the Turkish bread into four pieces and then lay flat and cut each piece in half, toasting until brown. Lay the toasted Turkish bread on a chopping board and smear both sides with hummus. Place 1 tablespoon of the tabouli over the hummus and gently press so it sticks.

Place the slices of cucumber and tomato on the base, then add the lamb patties and the red onion and top with some chilli sauce (optional). Top with baby English spinach and serve hot.

Funtastic Baby Facts

Newborns are covered in a waxy coating called vernix caseosa when then first make their grand entrance to the world.

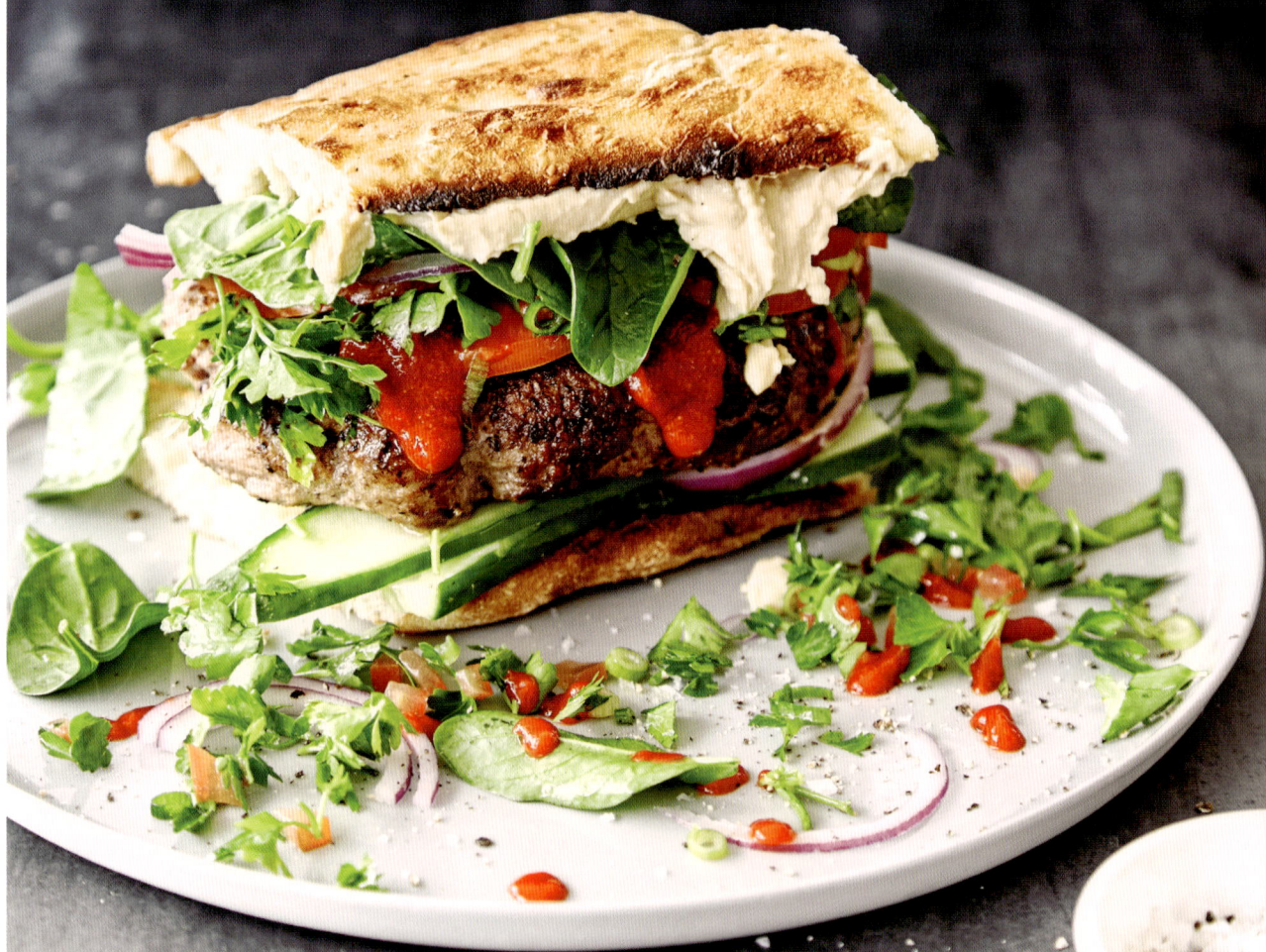

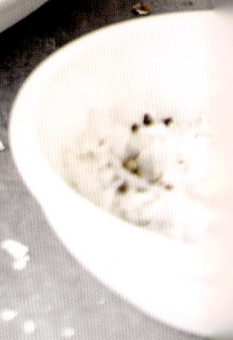

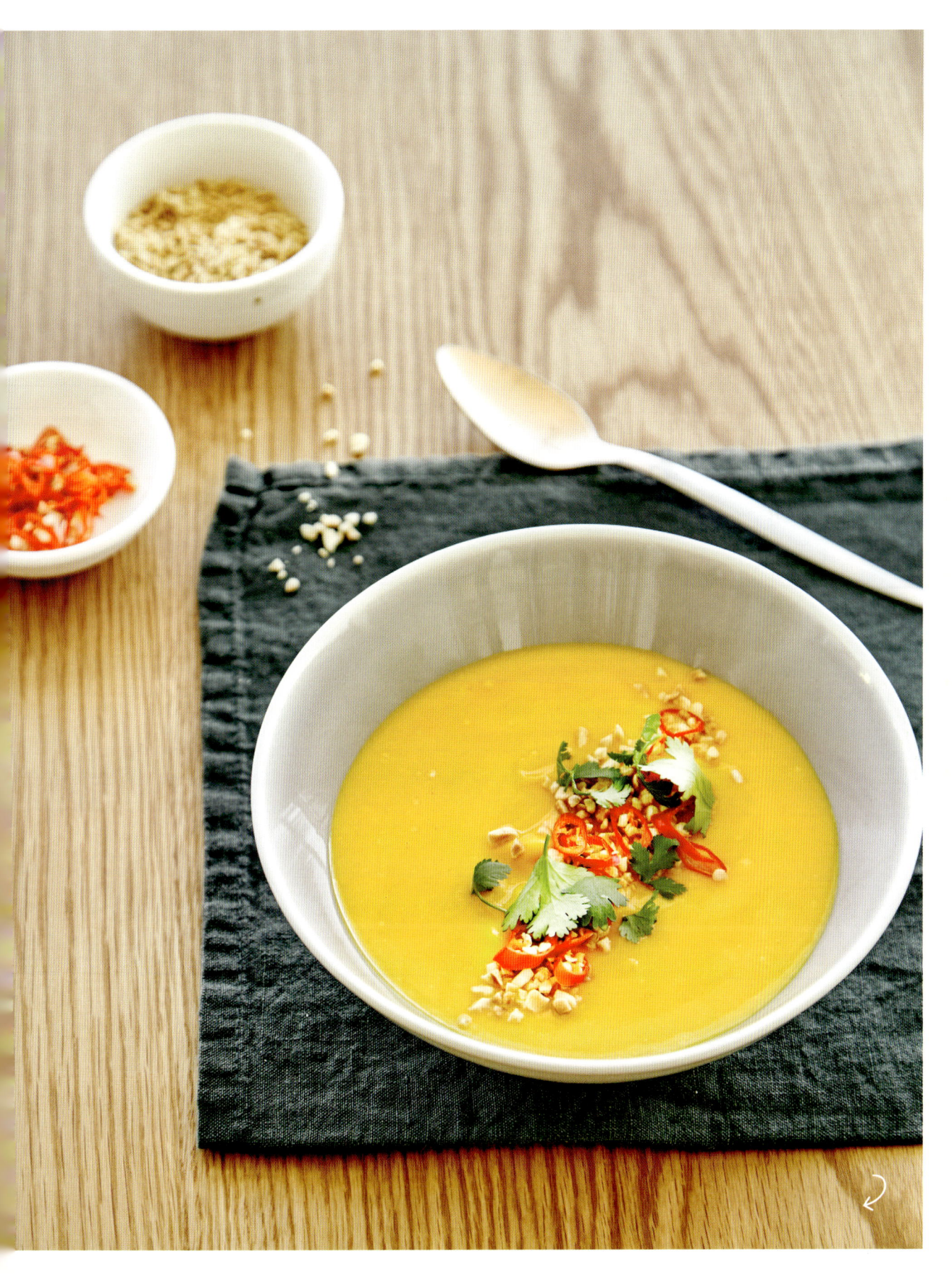

This is one of those dishes that you try once and then you have to have it again and again and again, it's just that good. Packed to the brim with sour, salty, sweet deliciousness from the roast pumpkin, coriander, coconut milk and lime the great thing about this soup is you can fortify it with some fish, prawns or chicken if you are looking for something a little heartier.

ROAST PUMPKIN & YELLOW CURRY SOUP

Serves 6
Cooking Time: 1 hour 20 minutes

INGREDIENTS

- × 2 tablespoons vegetable oil
- × 800 g (1 lb 12 oz) pumpkin (winter squash), roughly chopped
- × 1 carrot, roughly chopped
- × 1 onion, roughly chopped
- × 4 garlic cloves, unpeeled
- × 1 celery stalk, finely sliced
- × 1 lemongrass stalk (white part only), finely sliced
- × 25 g (1 oz) galangal (or ginger), julienned
- × 4 coriander (cilantro) roots, trimmed and finely chopped
- × 2 teaspoons yellow curry powder
- × 2 teaspoons turmeric

- × 2 tablespoons brown sugar
- × 1 litre (35 fl oz) chicken stock (see Basics, page 31 or unsalted if store-bought)
- × 400 ml (14 fl oz) coconut milk
- × 2 tablespoons fish sauce
- × 2 tablespoons light soy sauce
- × ½ lime, juiced
- × 6 teaspoons crushed peanuts, to garnish
- × 1 bunch baby bok choy (pak choy), roughly chopped
- × sea salt and cracked black pepper, to season
- × 1 long red chilli (optional), finely sliced
- × ¼ bunch coriander (cilantro), roughly chopped, to garnish

Preheat the oven to 180°C (350°F/Gas 4). Lightly grease a baking tray with a drizzle of vegetable oil.

Place the pumpkin, carrot and onion on the baking tray. Add the unpeeled garlic cloves and place the tray in the oven. Roast until the garlic is soft and the pumpkin and onion are browned. Remove from the oven and allow to cool slightly. Peel the garlic.

Heat 1 tablespoon of the vegetable oil in a large pot over medium heat. Add the celery, lemongrass, galangal and coriander root to the pot and fry until fragrant.

Add the yellow curry powder, turmeric and brown sugar and cook for a further 30 seconds.

Add the roast vegetables, chicken stock, coconut milk, fish sauce, light soy sauce, lime juice and bring the pot to a boil. Cover, reduce the heat to low and simmer for 30 minutes.

Remove the cover and simmer for a further 10 minutes. Remove the soup from the heat and allow to cool for 15 minutes.

Place a small, dry frying pan over medium heat and add the crushed peanuts. Cook until fragrant, then set aside the peanuts in a small bowl.

Using a blender, add the soup (make sure it is cool to avoid any mishaps) in small batches, puréeing until silky smooth and there are no lumps. Pour the soup into a clean saucepan and return it to the stove over low heat. Add the baby bok choy.

Taste the soup and season with salt and pepper, if it needs more sweet or sour flavour, add some brown sugar, lime juice or fish sauce to balance.

Serve the soup piping hot and garnished with sliced red chilli, crushed peanuts and coriander leaves.

From The Wise

Pizza is one dish that is almost always better when it's takeaway instead of homemade. The reason? Well aside from years of experience of churning out hundreds of pizzas a night, your local pizzeria also has superhot ovens that can generate the high temperatures required to create that puffy crusted, crisp based, gooey cheese deliciousness that gets even the most health conscience of us to salivate. So what are the alternatives if you want to make your own pizza at home? Well you can buy or build an oven for the backyard, get yourself a pizza stone or failing that a cast iron pan and the griller in the oven. I have used potatoes with rosemary and caramelized red onion as a topping but feel free to try a tomato with mozzarella and basil or any other combinations you can dream up.

POTATO & CARAMELIZED RED ONION PIZZA

Makes 2 pizzas
Cooking Time: 2 hours 45 minutes (don't worry, most of this time is waiting for the dough to rise!)

INGREDIENTS

PIZZA DOUGH

× 1 sachet dried yeast
× 1 tablespoon caster (superfine) sugar
× 420 g (15 oz) plain (all-purpose) flour, plus extra for dusting
× 1 teaspoon salt
× 4 tablespoons olive oil, plus extra for greasing the mixing bowl

× 2 desiree potatoes
× 1 red onion, thinly sliced
× 2 tablespoons balsamic vinegar
× 2 rosemary sprigs, leaves removed
× 130 g (4½ oz) mozzarella, grated
× 60 g (21/4 oz) parmesan cheese, shaved
× 2 tablespoons olive oil, plus extra to drizzle
× sea salt and cracked black pepper, to season

To make the pizza dough, add 1 sachet of instant yeast powder to a mixing bowl and add the caster sugar and 250 ml (9 fl oz) of warm water. Mix together and cover for 10 minutes. If it bubbles, the yeast is active if not, discard and start again.

Add the flour, salt and olive oil and combine well in the bowl until you have a rough dough.

Dust a clean work surface with flour and turn out the dough kneading for 8–10 minutes, the dough should be elastic and have a sheen to it. (If the dough is too wet add a little flour, if it is too dry wet your hands under the tap.)

Coat a mixing bowl in a drizzle of olive oil and add the dough, rubbing the exterior in olive oil before covering with a tea towel and allowing to rise for at least 2 hours.

Using a mandolin or a sharp knife, cut the potato into wafer-thin slices (the potato must be thin enough to see through or it will be still raw when the pizza is removed from the oven), then place in an airtight container.

Heat the olive oil in a frying pan over medium heat. When hot, add the onions and cook until they start to colour. Add the vinegar and cook until the onions caramelise. Remove from the pan and set aside.

About 20 minutes before you want to make your pizza, preheat the oven to its highest temperature or conversely put the grill on high and move the wire racks down so the pizza is in the centre of the oven. Add your pizza stone, cast iron pan or ovenproof frying pan.

When the dough has risen, punch it back down into a ball and turn it out on a lightly floured work surface and divide into two portions. Grab the first piece of dough and push it out to form a rough circle, then press out from the centre of the dough towards the edge with the heels of your palms stretching the dough out. Quarter turn and repeat until your pizza dough is a circular shape about the same size as the base of your pan or stone that is pre heating in the oven. Repeat with the other piece of dough.

Brush 1 tablespoon of olive oil over each pizza base. Scatter the caramelized onions, rosemary leaves, mozzarella and parmesan over the base. Top with the potatoes and season with sea salt and cracked black pepper.

Remove the pizza stone or pan from the oven and place on the stovetop. Carefully place one of the completed pizzas onto the stone or pan using a paddle and then return to the oven. Cook until the crusts are puffed up, mottled and slightly blackened and the cheese is melted (between 2-5 minutes), then remove from the oven carefully and slide the pizza onto a cutting board. Rest for 1–2 minutes and cut into slices. Repeat with the remaining pizza dough and toppings.

Like most things that are great in this world, this salad is very simple and yet totally delicious, so much so that I'm sure it will stay on the menu long after the little one is born. Packed with sweet roast pumpkin, fried haloumi, the nutty goodness of brown rice and chickpeas, the freshness of mint, coriander and cucumber, the tang of lemon and the creamy deliciousness of hummus this dish is really easy to throw together when you don't have a lot of time on your hands but want to make a nutritious, tasty dinner.

BROWN RICE SALAD WITH PUMPKIN, CHICKPEAS & HALOUMI

Serves 4
Cooking Time: 40 minutes

INGREDIENTS

- × 2 tablespoons olive oil, plus extra for drizzling
- × 250 g (9 oz) pumpkin (winter squash), cut into cubes
- × 1 capsicum (pepper), cut lengthways
- × 200 g (7 oz) brown rice
- × 180 g (6½ oz) haloumi cheese, sliced
- × zest and juice of ½ lemon
- × 2 tablespoons red wine vinegar
- × 400 g (14 oz) tinned chickpeas, drained
- × ¼ bunch mint, roughly chopped
- × ½ bunch coriander (cilantro), roughly chopped
- × sea salt and cracked black pepper, to season
- × 100 g (3½ oz) rocket (arugula)
- × 75 g (3 oz) cherry tomatoes, roughly chopped
- × 1 Lebanese (short) cucumber, thinly sliced lengthways
- × 4 heaped tablespoons hummus (see Basics, page 36 or use store-bought)

Preheat the oven to 180˚C (350˚F/Gas 4). Lightly grease a baking tray with a drizzle of olive oil.

Add the pumpkin and capsicum to the baking tray. Place the tray in the oven and cook until the pumpkin is roasted and the skin of the capsicum is black and mottled. Remove the baking tray from the oven and place the capsicum in a plastic bag, tying the end and allowing the heat to sweat the skin. Remove the capsicum from the bag and peel off the skin, slice into thin strips and set aside.

Meanwhile, place the rice in a rice cooker and cover with 400 ml (14 fl oz) water and cook until done OR place rice in a saucepan and cover with 800 ml (28 fl oz) water and bring to the boil. Reduce the heat to a simmer and cook for about 20 minutes, or until the water is absorbed and rice is tender yet firm. Turn off the rice, or remove from the heat, and leave to stand in steam for 10 minutes, then remove and spread over a baking tray to cool.

Heat a drizzle of olive oil in a non-stick frying pan over medium heat. When hot, add the haloumi and cook till brown, then set aside on a paper towel to drain.

Add the rice to a large mixing bowl with the lemon zest and juice. Add 1 tablespoon of olive oil and 1 tablespoon of red wine vinegar. Add the pumpkin, capsicum, chickpeas, mint coriander and haloumi and gently mix to combine. Season with salt and cracked black pepper and set aside.

Add the rocket, tomato and cucumber to a separate mixing bowl. Dress with the remaining olive oil and red wine vinegar, season with salt and pepper and toss.

Serve the rice with a heaped tablespoon of hummus and top with the rocket, cherry tomatoes and cucumber.

Funtastic Baby Facts
Did you know the first poop your little one will do is called meconium?

When I was a kid, potato and leek soup was one of the favourite dishes that my mother made, in fact on a cold winter's day there was nothing better than a hot bowl of that buttery, luxurious, luscious, creamy, velvety soup. Now this update is nothing on the original, it's a classic for a reason but the roasted vegetables and mustard do give it an interesting and delicious twist.

POTATO, LEEK & CAULIFLOWER SOUP WITH ENGLISH MUSTARD

Serves 6
Cooking Time: 1 hour 15 minutes

INGREDIENTS

× ½ white onion, roughly chopped
× 1 carrot, roughly chopped
× 5 garlic cloves, unpeeled
× 1 small cauliflower
× 1 tablespoon unsalted butter
× 1 tablespoon olive oil, plus extra for drizzling
× 1 leek, thinly sliced
× 1 thyme sprig, leaves finely chopped

× 1 celery stalk, with leaves on, chopped
× 2 potatoes, chopped
× 1 teaspoon English mustard
× 6 slices prosciutto
× 1 litre (35 fl oz) chicken stock (see Basics, page 31 or unsalted if using store-bought)
× sea salt and cracked black pepper, to season

METHOD

Preheat the oven to 180°C (350°F/Gas 4). Grease a baking tray with a drizzle of olive oil.

Add the onion, carrot and garlic cloves to the baking tray. Break the florets from the stem of the cauliflower and place on the baking tray. Drizzle the vegetables liberally with olive oil and roast in the oven until browned, turning when needed. Remove from the oven and leave to cool slightly. Peel the garlic.

Heat the butter and oil in a pot over medium heat. Add the leeks and thyme, frying over low heat until soft. Add the celery and potatoes and cook for a further 10 minutes. Add the oven-roasted vegetables and garlic to the pot, with the English mustard and the chicken stock.

Bring to the boil, then reduce to a simmer, cooking for 30 minutes with the lid off. Season with salt and cracked black pepper. Remove from the heat and leave to cool for 10 minutes on the stovetop. When the soup has cooled a little, pour a small batch in a blender (ensuring not to fill past halfway) and purée until smooth. Set aside in a clean bowl and repeat with the rest of the soup. Return the soup to the stovetop and reheat.

Heat some olive oil in a frying pan over medium heat. When hot, add the prosciutto and brown on one side then turn and brown the other side. Remove the prosciutto from the pan and place on paper towels to drain.

To serve, pour the soup into each bowl and top with some finely sliced prosciutto crumbled over the top.

Funtastic Baby Facts

Did you know that newborns don't cry tears? They are born with basal tearing which creates enough moisture to keep the eyes wet and healthy. The real tears begin later!

There are almost as many variations of this soup as there are ramen restaurants in Japan. In fact, this dish is so popular you can not only experience in the multitude of different regional varieties on offer in Japan and around the world but also buy it pre-packaged or in canned in tins, visit the ramen museum or watch the several full-length feature films made about these delicious noodles.

I have chosen a poultry version with soy chicken and egg but you can add a variety of healthy ingredients to it which are great for both mother and baby.

CHICKEN & EGG RAMEN

Serves 4

Cooking Time: 50 minutes

INGREDIENTS

SOY CHICKEN
- × 3 tablespoons dark soy
- × 1tablespoons light soy
- × 1 teaspoon sesame oil
- × 4 chicken thighs

SOUP
- × 750 ml (26 fl oz) chicken stock (see Basics, 31 or unsalted if using store-bought)
- × 3 tablespoons white miso paste

- × 3 tablespoons light soy
- × 6 shitake mushrooms, thinly sliced
- × 4 eggs
- × 125 g (4½ oz) ramen noodles
- × 50 g (13/4 oz) silken tofu, cut into cubes
- × 50 g (13/4 oz) bok choy (pak choy), cut into thin strips
- × 25 g (1 oz) nori, cut into thin strips
- × 2 spring onions, thinly sliced
- × 25 g (1 oz) fresh peeled ginger, julienned

To make the soy chicken, add the dark soy, light soy and sesame oil to a mixing bowl and combine. Add chicken and coat well, then leave to marinate in the fridge for a minimum of 30 minutes.

Heat the chicken stock in a saucepan and bring to the boil. Add the white miso paste, soy sauce and mushrooms and reduce the heat to a simmer.

Bring another saucepan of water to a rolling boil and add the eggs. Cook until hard-boiled then remove from the water, then set aside to cool. Peel and cut in half.

Heat a drizzle of vegetable oil in a frying pan over medium heat. Add the chicken thighs and cook, checking regularly, until they are sticky and caramelised on one side, then flip over and repeat until both sides are done and the chicken is fully cooked through (check by slicing one in half, if it is a little under just return it to the pan). Place the cooked chicken on a plate and set aside to cool. Slice the chicken into thin strips.

Add the noodles, tofu, bok choy and nori to the simmering dashi soup and cook for 2 minutes.

To serve, add the noddles to each bowl and top with the sliced chicken and eggs. Ladle the soup mix over the noodles, making sure each serving gets the mushrooms, tofu, bok choy and nori. Garnish with the spring onions and fresh sliced ginger.

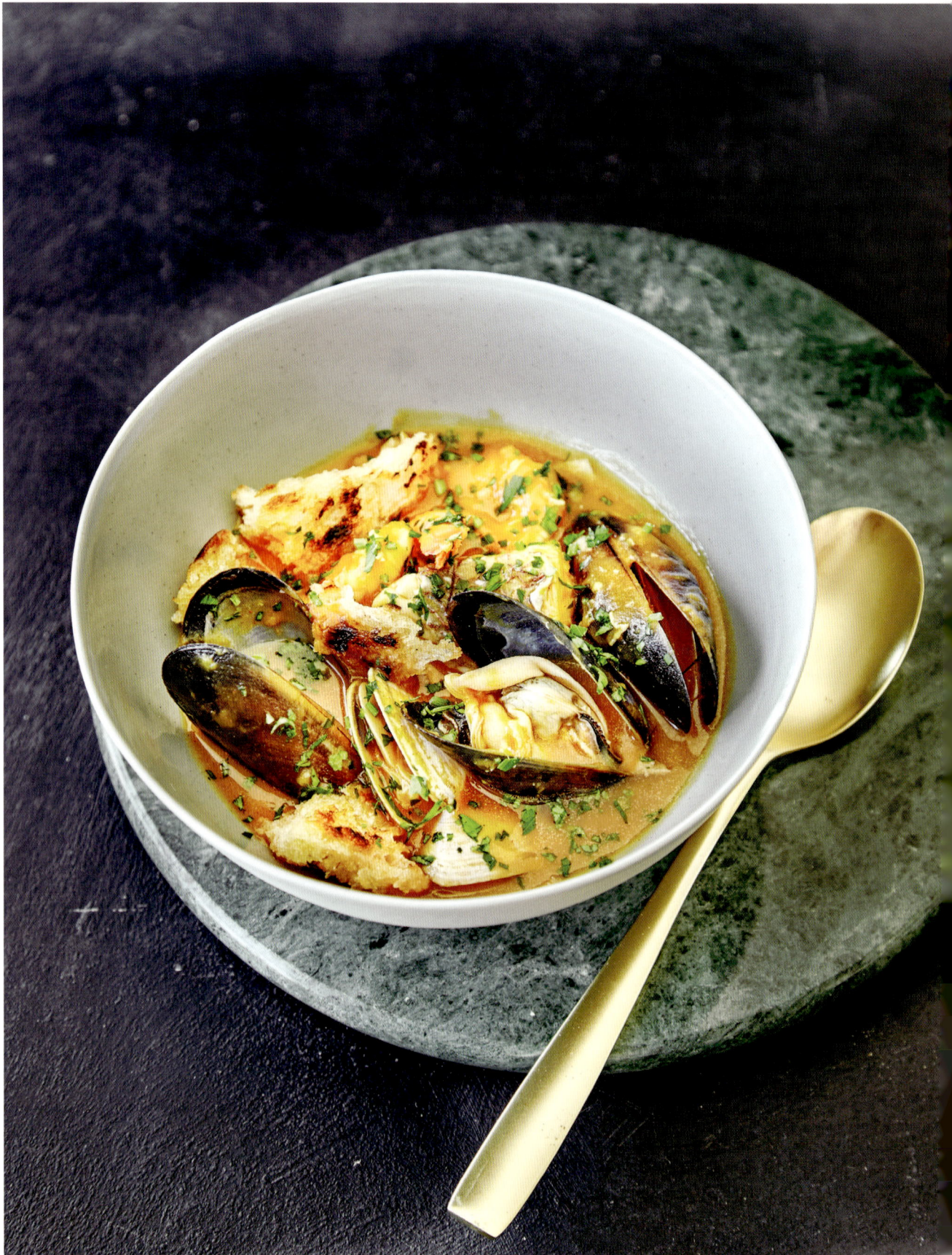

This a classic seafood stew packed with prawns, mussels, clams and snapper. Just remember that while fish is high in those valuable omega-3 fatty acids that a mother and unborn child need, you need to make sure that you limit your fish intake to 2–3 serves per week (or only once of you are eating catfish, deep sea perch, flake or marlin) as it can contain mercury. As for the clams and mussels, remember the golden rule when cooking them: you don't open your mouth for them if they don't open theirs.

FISH STEW

Serves 6
Cooking Time: 1 hour 55 minutes

INGREDIENTS

- × 2 garlic cloves, roughly chopped
- × ½ onion, roughly chopped
- × 2 carrots, roughly chopped
- × ½ green capsicum (pepper), roughly chopped
- × 1 celery stalk, leaves on, roughly chopped
- × 2 basil sprigs, chopped
- × 2 oregano sprigs, chopped
- × 2 continental parsley sprigs, chopped, plus extra to garnish
- × 1 teaspoon ground black pepper
- × 2 teaspoons smoked paprika
- × 1 teaspoon of tabasco sauce
- × 1 tablespoon red wine vinegar
- × 1 tablespoon Worcestershire sauce
- × 3 x 400 g (14 oz) tinned crushed tomatoes
- × 1 litre (35 fl oz) of fish stock (see Basics, page 33 or unsalted if using store-bought)
- × 12 mussels, scrubbed and de-bearded
- × 12 clams, scrubbed
- × 250 g (9 oz) snapper, cut into 12 bite-sized chunks
- × 12 prawns (shrimp), peeled and deveined (reserving the heads and shells)
- × sea salt, to season

METHOD

Heat some olive oil in a pot over medium heat. Add the garlic and chopped vegetables, sautéing until soft. Add the basil, oregano, parsley, black pepper, smoked paprika, tabasco, red wine vinegar and Worcestershire sauce. Add the crushed tomatoes and stir well. Bring the liquid to the boil, then reduce the heat to low. Cover and simmer for 30 minutes. Remove the lid and stir well, simmering for another 15 minutes. Remove the pot from the heat and allow the liquid to cool for about 20 minutes.

Continued ↘

MORE SUBSTANTIAL

FISH STEW CONTINUED...

Add a small batch of the cooled liquid into a blender (careful not to fill past halfway) and purée until there are no lumps. Remove and place the liquid into mixing bowl. Repeat until all the soup base is puréed.

Heat the fish stock in a large pot over medium heat and bring to a simmer. Add the soup base to the pot, stir well and bring to a boil. Reduce the heat to a simmer for 10 minutes.

Add the mussels and clams and cook for 10 minutes. Add the fish and the prawns (shrimp) and cook for a further 5 minutes. Remove the pot from the heat and discard any of the mussels and clams that have not opened. Season with salt and pepper.

Divide the seafood between the bowls so everyone gets two pieces of everything and ladle the soup over. Garnish with some parsley and a drizzle of olive oil.

This is one of those great share dishes you can make on a warm summer's day while you're sitting around the barbecue in the afternoon sun with friends. The fresh, crisp flavours of the mint yoghurt go perfectly with the smoky sweet lamb and tangy couscous. Serve of the pita bread and a big bowl of tabouli.

LAMB SHISH KEBAB WITH MINT YOGHURT & CHICKPEA SPINACH COUSCOUS

Serves 4

Cooking Time: 1 hour 25 minutes.

INGREDIENTS

LAMB SHISH KEBAB

- × ¼ teaspoon cumin
- × ¼ teaspoon cinnamon
- × ¼ teaspoon smoked paprika
- × ¼ teaspoon ground coriander
- × ¼ teaspoon crushed black pepper
- × ¼ teaspoon sea salt
- × ¼ teaspoon nutmeg
- × ¼ teaspoon dried oregano
- × ½ onion, roughly chopped
- × ¼ bunch flat-leaf (Italian) parsley, roughly chopped
- × 500 g (1 lb 2 oz) minced (ground) lamb
- × 2 tablespoons olive oil

MINT YOGHURT

- × ½ Lebanese (short) cucumber, coarsely grated
- × ¼ bunch mint, leaves finely chopped
- × 125 g (4½ oz) Greek-style yoghurt
- × juice of ¼ of a lemon
- × sea salt and cracked black pepper, to season

CHICKPEA SPINACH COUSCOUS

- × 300 ml (101/2 fl oz) chicken stock (see Basics, page 31 or unsalted if using store-bought)
- × 3 garlic cloves, crushed
- × 2 teaspoons cumin
- × 2 teaspoons smoked paprika
- × 200 g (7 oz) couscous
- × ½ red onion, thinly sliced
- × 2 spring onions (scallions), thinly sliced
- × ½ bunch flat-leaf (Italian) parsley, roughly chopped
- × 3 tomatoes, deseeded and diced
- × 1 Lebanese (short) cucumber, thinly sliced lengthways
- × 400 g (14 oz) tinned chickpeas
- × 150 g (5½ oz) baby English spinach
- × juice of ½ a lemon
- × 2 tablespoons olive oil
- × sea salt and cracked black pepper, to season

Continued ⤵

MORE SUBSTANTIAL

LAMB SHISH KEBAB WITH MINT YOGHURT & CHICKPEA SPINACH COUSCOUS CONTINUED...

To make the lamb shish kebab, place a dry frying pan over low heat and add the cumin, cinnamon, smoked paprika, ground coriander, crushed black pepper, sea salt, nutmeg and dried oregano. Cook until fragrant, then remove the spice mix from the heat, setting aside in a small bowl.

Add the onion and parsley to a food processor and blend until they form a paste with no large chunks. Add the lamb, spice mix and the olive oil to the onions in the food processor and pulse until combined.

If you are using bamboo skewers, soak them in boiling water for 30 minutes beforehand.

Break the lamb up into even portions (should form about 8-10 shish kebab, depending on the size) and mould one at a time to form a sausage shape. Press the skewer through gently and repeat with the rest of the meat. Set aside in the fridge for 1 hour.

To make the mint yoghurt, add the cucumber and mint leaves to a small mixing bowl. Spoon in the yoghurt, squeeze in the lemon juice and season with salt and pepper. Mix together well, cover and refrigerate until needed.

To make the chickpea spinach couscous first bring the chicken stock to the boil. Add the garlic, cumin and smoked paprika and simmer for 5 minutes.

Add the couscous to a heatproof bowl, pour over the chicken stock and let steep until all the stock is absorbed (about 5-10 minutes).

Add the red onion, spring onions and parsley to a bowl. Add the tomato and cucumber and gently mix to combine. Set aside until needed.

Remove the lamb shish kebabs from the fridge and heat the barbecue hotplate or chargrill pan to medium. Place the lamb shish kebabs on the barbecue and cook for about 4-5 minutes per side, then remove from the heat to rest for a few minutes (check first to ensure the meat is fully cooked through).

Remove the garlic from the couscous. Add the tomatoes, parsley and onion, then the chickpeas and baby English spinach. Toss together well, drizzle over the olive oil and lemon juice, season with salt and pepper and toss.

To serve, add a generous amount of the couscous to each plate, top with two lamb shish kebabs and cover with several tablespoons of the mint yoghurt.

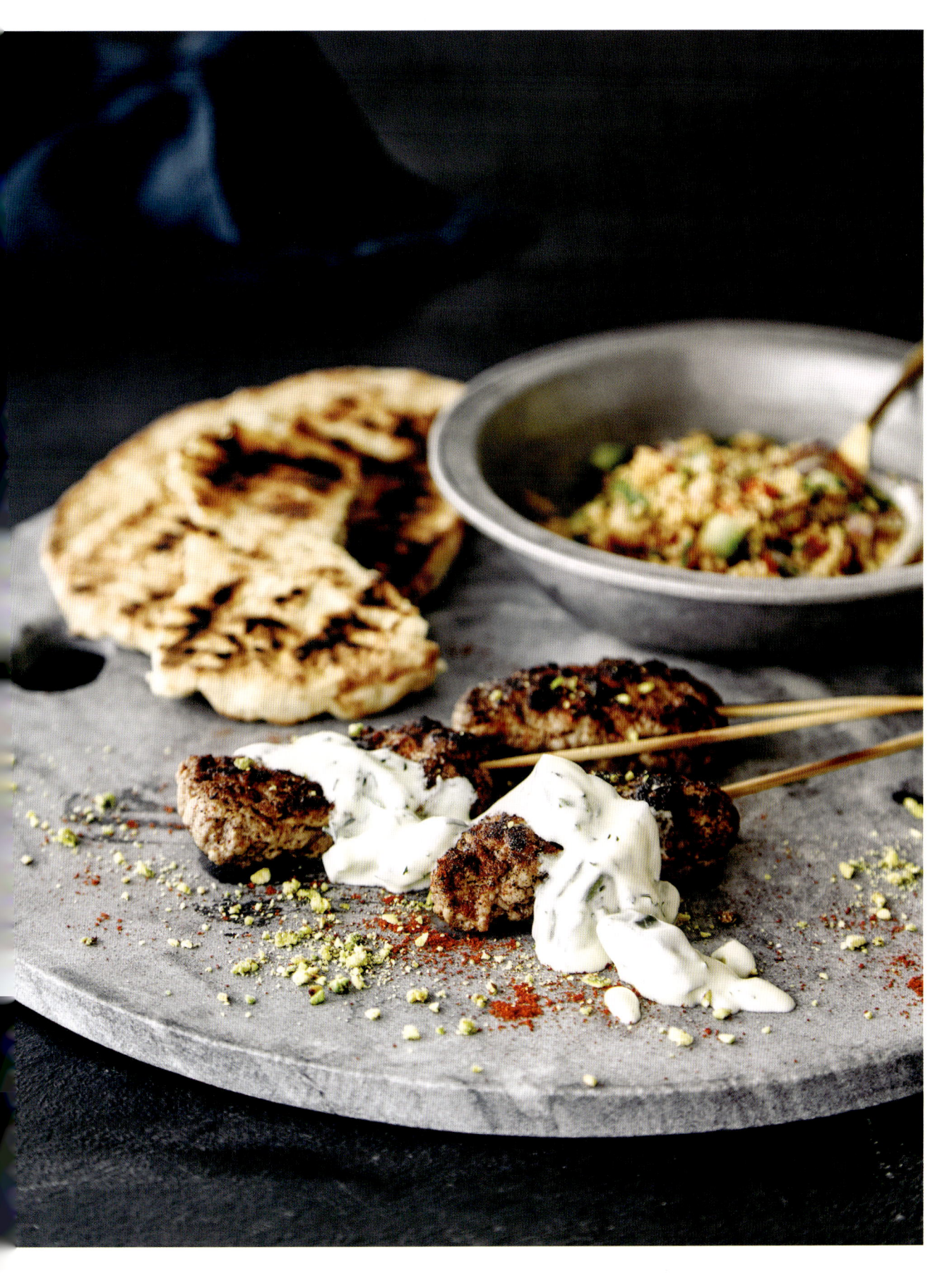

This dish is a family favourite and because you can really go to town on the choy sum it's an excellent meal to make for your pregnant partner as a bit of a treat and still get those prized folates, as well as iron and omega-3 fatty acids from the prawns (just ensure you cook them through fully).

CHAR KWAY TEOW

Serves 6
Cooking Time: 30 minutes

INGREDIENTS

- × 600 g (21 oz) fresh flat rice noodles
- × 2 tablespoons cooking caramel (karamel masakan)
- × 2 tablespoons light soy sauce
- × 1 tablespoon fish sauce
- × 1 teaspoon dark sugar
- × 3 eggs
- × 25 g (1 oz) ginger, julienned
- × 2 garlic cloves, crushed
- × 2 tablespoons chilli sambal (see Basics, page 34) or chilli, lemongrass and ginger mix (see page 110), optional
- × ¾ onion, thinly sliced
- × 12 prawns (shrimp), peeled and deveined or 10 prawn cakes (see page 110), sliced
- × 200 g (7 oz) char siu, thinly sliced
- × 1 bunch choy sum, chopped
- × 1 lime, halved
- × 1/2 bunch coriander (cilantro), roughly chopped
- × 2 spring onions, finely chopped

Cut the rice noodles into thick slices and separate them by hand, setting aside in a mixing bowl.

Place the cooking caramel, light soy sauce, fish sauce and dark sugar in a bowl and mix well. Crack the eggs into a bowl and whisk together.

Place a wok over medium heat and add a drizzle of vegetable oil. When hot, add the eggs and cook until the bottom is browned. Flip one side of the omelette over the other and cook under egg is fully set. Remove from pan and roughly chop setting aside till later.

Wipe the wok clean and place back over medium heat. Add a drizzle of vegetable oil and when smoking hot, add the ginger, garlic and if using, either the chilli sambal or the chilli, lemongrass and ginger mix and stir. Add the onions and prawns (or prawn cakes), frying until the prawns are fully cooked through.

Add the char siu, egg omelette, choy sum and stir well. Add the noodles and the cooking caramel mixture, then squeeze both lime halves over the top and stir from the bottom.

Cook for a 1–2 minutes, or until the noodles are soft, then add the coriander and the spring onions. Remove from the heat and serve.

Funtastic Baby Facts

Did you know it's not that uncommon for a newborn to have a coating of downy hair over their bodies called lanugo? It normally disappears in a few days or a week.

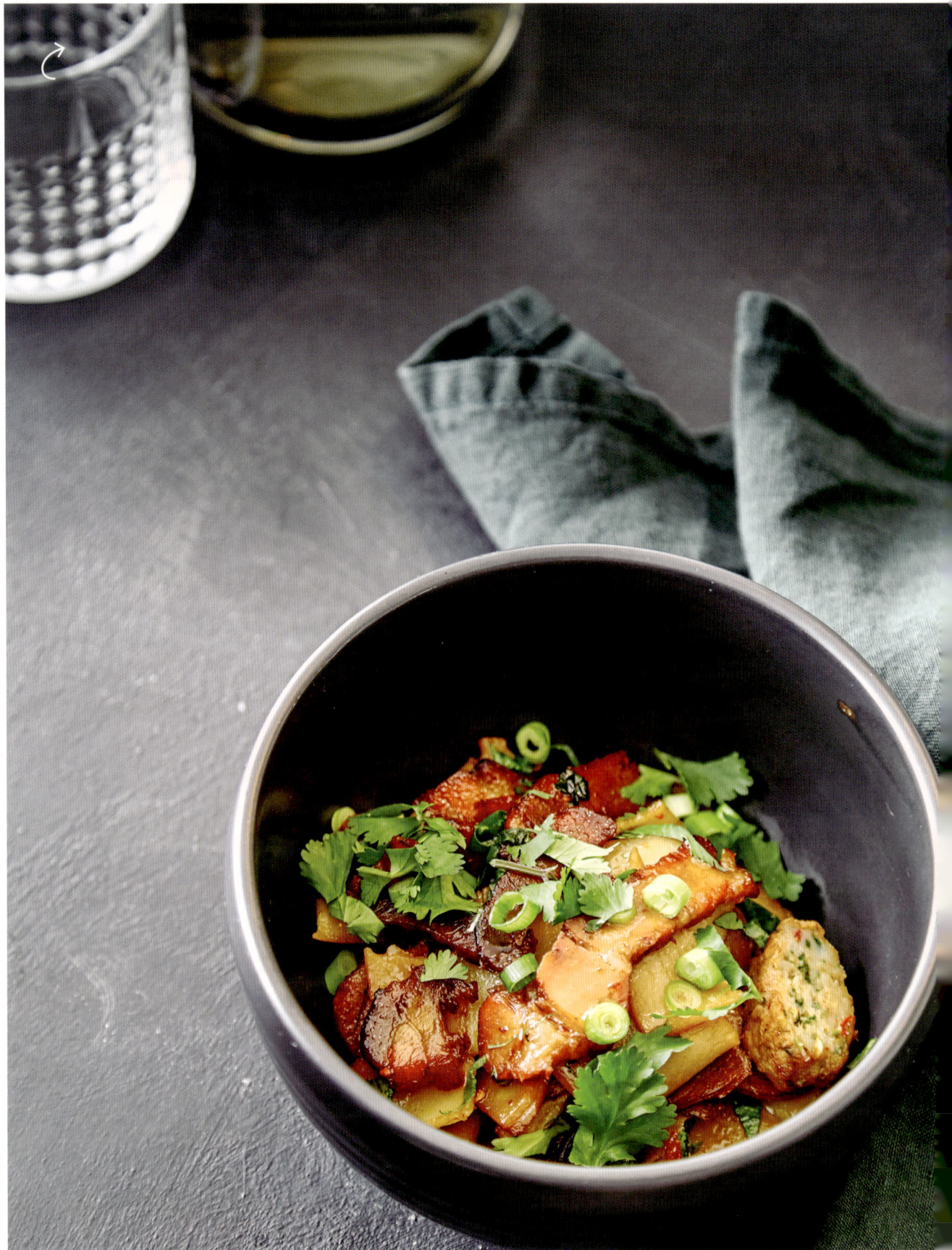

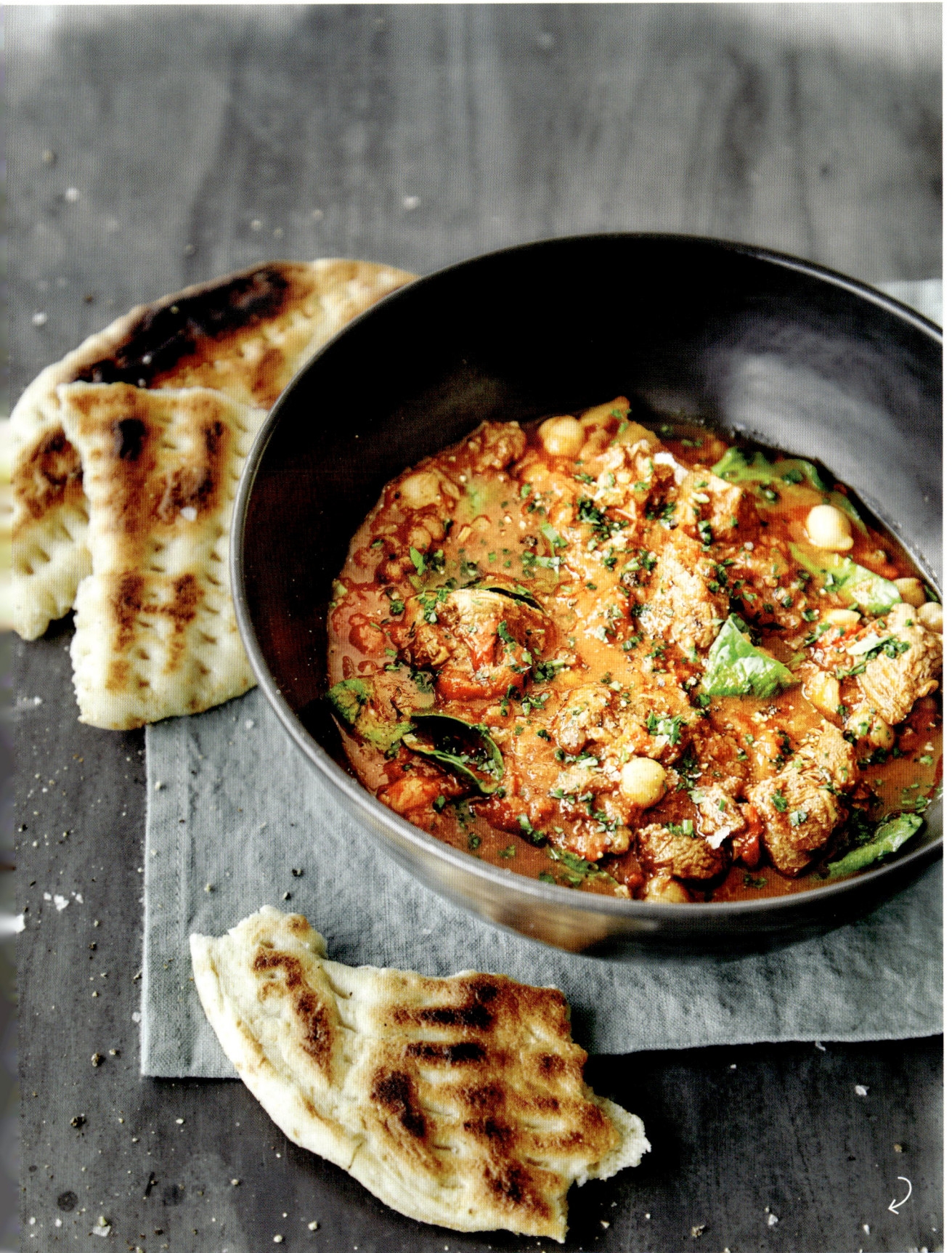

Sometimes when it's cold outside all you want to do is curl up on the couch with a big bowl of comfort food and relax in front of the TV. If you want a bowl of delicious comfort food, then you don't have to look much further than this Moroccan-style lamb stew with chickpeas, lentils and spinach.

MOROCCAN LAMB STEW WITH CHICKPEAS & LENTILS

Serves 6
Cooking Time: 2 hours 30 minutes

INGREDIENTS

MOROCCAN SPICE MIX
× 1 tablespoon cumin
× 2 tablespoons smoked paprika
× ½ teaspoon ground coriander
× ½ tablespoon cracked black pepper
× ½ teaspoon cinnamon
× ½ teaspoon allspice
× ¼ teaspoon ground clove
× 1 tablespoon sea salt

× 1 onion, halved
× 4 garlic cloves, unpeeled

× 1 kg (2 lb 4 oz) lamb shoulder
× 1 tablespoon sea salt
× 1/2 lemon
× 2 tablespoons tomato paste (concentrated purée)
× 1 litre (35 fl oz) beef stock
× 800 g (1 lb 12 oz) tinned crushed tomatoes
× 400 g (14 oz) tinned chickpeas, drained
× 400 g (14 oz) tinned brown lentils, drained
× 70 g (2 ½ oz) baby English spinach
× ¾ bunch coriander (cilantro), roughly chopped
× 6 tablespoons thick Greek-style yoghurt, to serve

Preheat oven to 190°C (375°F/Gas 5). Grease a baking tray.

To make the Moroccan spice mix, add the cumin, smoked paprika, ground coriander, cracked black pepper, cinnamon, allspice and ground clove to a small dry frying pan and place over low heat, cooking until fragrant. Place the cooked spices into a small bowl, add the sea salt and set aside until later.

Place the onion and unpeeled garlic on a baking tray and roast until the garlic is soft and the onion is roasted and blackened. Remove from the oven, peel the garlic and roughly chop, setting aside until later.

Roughly chop the lamb into bite-sized chunks and season with 1 tablespoon of sea salt. Zest the lemon into a bowl, making sure to avoid the white pith and then juice what remains.

Drizzle the olive oil into a frying pan over medium heat and add the lamb, searing on all sides until brown. Add the tomato paste to the pan and stir well. Add the spice mix to the seared lamb and stir well, mixing everything together and frying for about 30 seconds more, then Remove from the heat and place on an unused burner at the back of the stove.

Drizzle the olive oil in a large pot over medium heat and add the roasted garlic and onions. Add the seared lamb to the pot then place the frying pan back over a low flame and deglaze with a cup of the beef stock, ensuring you scrape up all the browned meat and blacked spice from the bottom of the pan with a wooden spoon.

Pour the liquid into the pot. Add the remaining beef stock, tomatoes, lemon zest, lemon juice, chickpeas and lentils to the pot. Cover, bring to the boil and then reduce to a low simmer, cooking for 1 hour.

After 1 hour, remove the lid and cook for a further 1 hour, stirring every 15 minutes. (You will know when dish is cooked because the meat will be tender and fall apart.) Turn off the heat and add the spinach, stirring through.

Add the coriander to the pot (leaving a couple of tablespoons for garnish) stirring through. Taste and season salt and black pepper.

Serve with 1 tablespoon of the Greek-style yoghurt on the top of each dish and garnish with coriander. This stew goes great with brown rice, pearl couscous or toasted wholemeal pita bread to mop it up.

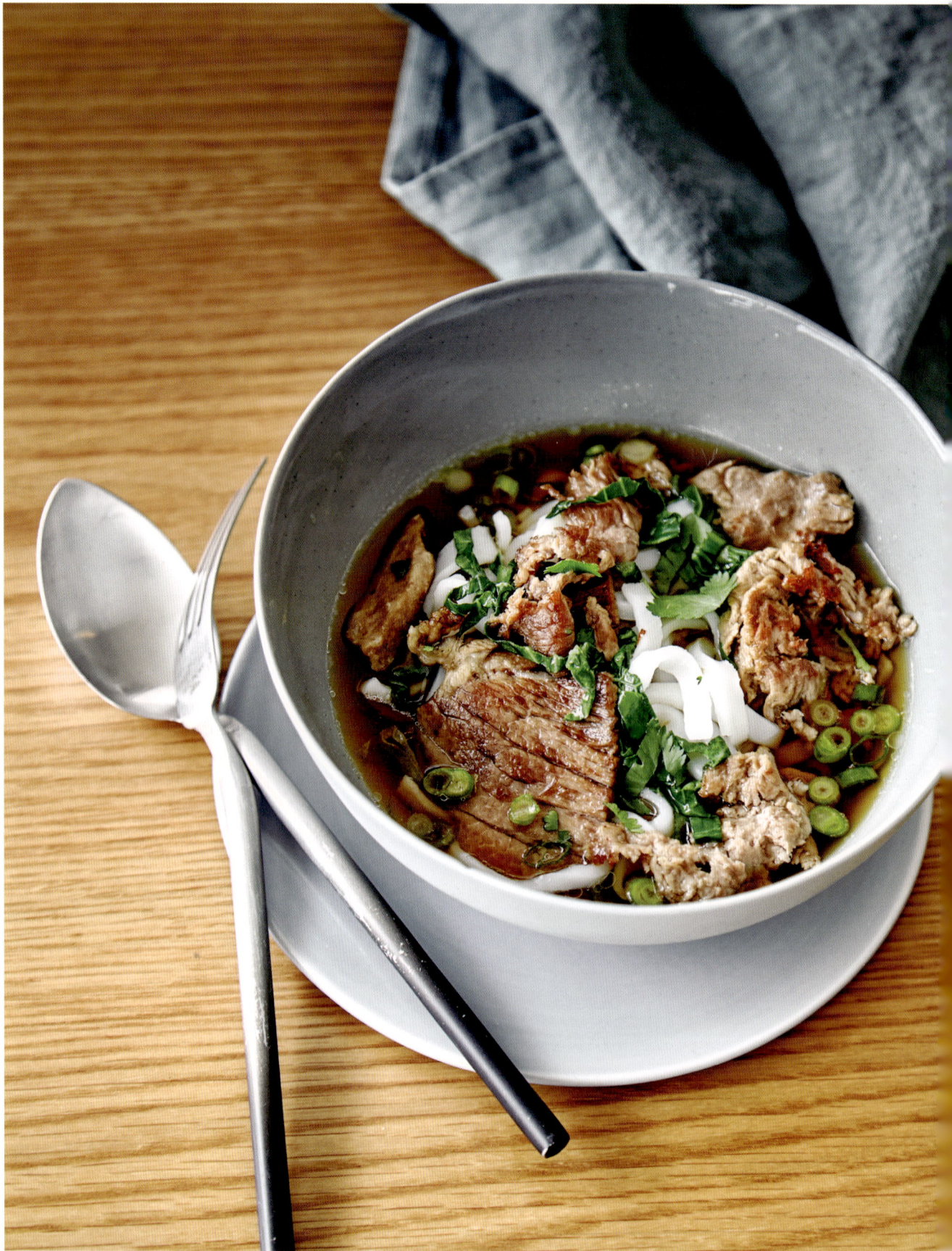

To make this pregnancy friendly version we have had to make a few minor changes by omitting the raw sirloin and sprouts that are normally poached in the soup by the hot broth. Luckily these changes don't make a huge difference and we have lost none of the wonderful and dark rich flavours that make this soup so unforgettably delicious. To make this dish you will need some clean muslin cloth.

BEEF PHO

Serves 6
Cooking Time: 2 hours 45 minutes

INGREDIENTS

- × 5 star anise
- × 3 pieces of cassia bark (or 1 quill cinnamon will do)
- × 1 teaspoon fennel seeds
- × 5 cloves
- × 10 black peppercorns
- × 2 black cardamom pods (also known as tsao-ko or thảo quả)
- × 400 g (14 oz) beef brisket
- × 2 onions
- × 4 garlic cloves, unpeeled
- × 2 litres (70 fl oz) beef stock (see Basics, page 32 or unsalted if using store-bought)

- × 50 g (13/4 oz) ginger
- × 3 tablespoons fish sauce
- × 3 tablespoons light soy sauce
- × 1 tablespoon brown sugar
- × juice of 1/2 a lime
- × 300 g (10½ oz) dried rice stick noodles
- × 1 bunch gai lan or choy sum, roughly chopped
- × 2 spring onion (scallion) stalks, finely sliced
- × ¼ bunch coriander (cilantro), finely sliced
- × sea salt, to season

METHOD

Preheat the oven to 180°C (350°F/Gas 4). Grease a baking tray with a drizzle of vegetable oil.

Place a small frying pan over medium heat and add the star anise, cassia bark, fennel seeds, cloves, black peppercorns and black cardamom pods, cooking until fragrant. Remove the spices from the heat and crush using a mortar and pestle or cover them in a tea towel and crush with a rolling pin.

Cut a square of muslin cloth, run it under some water then wring it out. Place the spices inside and tie securely so they won't escape when submerged in the stock.

Remove beef brisket from the fridge and sprinkle with sea salt.

(continued)

BEEF PHO CONTINUED...

Place 2 whole onions and the unpeeled garlic on the tray. Roast in the oven until the garlic is soft and the onion is mottled brown and blackened.

Place a pot over low heat and pour in the beef stock.

Place a cast iron pan over medium heat and drizzle with a little vegetable oil. When hot, carefully put the beef brisket in and brown on all sides, then add to the pot with the beef stock. Add the blackened onion and garlic, the ginger and the muslin cloth with the spices. Bring the pot to the boil, cover and reduce the heat to low and simmer for 1 hour. Remove the lid and simmer for a further 1 hour.

Once the soup has finished simmering, grab some tongs and fish out the brisket, placing it on a chopping board to cool.

Set a sieve over a large bowl and carefully strain the soup.

Clean the pot and pour the soup back in, then place it over medium heat. Thinly slice the brisket and add to the pot. Add the fish sauce, light soy sauce, brown sugar and lime juice to the pot and stir. Add the dried rice stick noodles and cook until soft. Add the gai lan and stir through then remove the pot from heat.

To serve, use the tongs to place an even amount of noodles in each bowl then add the beef brisket. Pour the soup into each bowl and serve garnished with spring onion and coriander.

It is totally acceptable if you want to use store-bought red curry paste and skip making your own, but I implore you to make a batch of the chilli sambal to have in your refrigerator. It is not only incredible in this dish; it's great to use as a base for stir fries or just as a condiment to spice up a sandwich.

BAKED RED CURRY WITH PORK & SAMBAL MEATBALLS

Serves 6
Cooking Time: 2 hours 20 minutes

INGREDIENTS

MEATBALLS
× 70 g (2½ oz) long grain rice
× 500 g (1 lb 2 oz) beef chuck, chopped
× 500 g (1 lb 2 oz) pork fillets, chopped
× 25 g (1 oz) ginger, grated
× 4 garlic cloves
× 2 tablespoons chilli sambal (see Basics, page 34 or store-bought if you prefer)
× 2 tablespoons fish sauce
× 2 tablespoons light soy sauce
× 70 g (2½ oz) plain (all-purpose) flour, to dust meatballs
× 3 tablespoons vegetable oil, for frying

BAKED RED CURRY
× 2 tablespoons red curry paste (see Basics, page 35 or store-bought if you prefer)
× 4 garlic cloves, sliced
× 3 onions, sliced
× 30g (1 oz) ginger, grated
× 1 long red chilli, sliced
× 2 tablespoons fish sauce
× 2 tablespoons light soy sauce
× 800 ml (28 fl oz) coconut milk
× 1 tablespoon palm sugar
× juice of 1 lime
× 40 g (1½ oz) Thai basil, chopped
× 1 bunch choy sum, chopped
× coriander (cilantro) leaves, finely chopped, to garnish

Continued ⤵

MORE SUBSTANTIAL

BAKED RED CURRY WITH PORK & SAMBAL MEATBALLS CONTINUED...

Preheat the oven to 180˚C (350˚F/Gas 4).

Place the rice in a rice cooker and cover with 70 ml (2½ fl oz) water and cook until done OR place rice in a saucepan, cover with 140 ml (43/4 fl oz) of water and bring to the boil. Reduce the heat to a simmer and cook for 10–15 minutes or until the water is absorbed and rice is tender yet firm. Leave to stand in the steam for 10 minutes, then remove the rice and spread over a baking tray to cool.

To make the meatballs, place the beef, pork, ginger, garlic, chilli sambal, fish sauce and light soy into a food processor and blend. (Do this in batches if your food processor is too small.) Blend the meatball mixture until it is a smooth paste with no chunks and transfer to a large mixing bowl. Add the rice to the meat and combine well.

Place the flour onto a large plate. Scoop out a heaped tablespoon of the mixture and form into a ball between the palms of your hands. Place the meatball onto the floured plated and roll around until covered, then set aside on a baking tray. Repeat this process until all the meat mixture is used.

Heat the vegetable oil in a deep frying pan or wok over medium heat. When the oil is hot, fry the meatballs in batches until golden brown, leaving to drain on paper towels.

To make the baked red curry, place the red curry paste in a dry frying pan over medium heat and cook until fragrant. Add the mixture to a bowl. Add the garlic, onion, ginger, long red chilli to the mixing bowl. Add the fish sauce, light soy sauce, coconut milk, palm sugar and lime juice to the bowl and mix well.

Place the meatballs in a clay pot or casserole dish and pour the coconut mixture over the top. Cover and cook in the oven for 1 hour. Add the Thai basil and choy sum, stirring through. Cover and return to oven for a further 30 minutes. Remove the curry from the oven, garnish with coriander and serve with steamed rice.

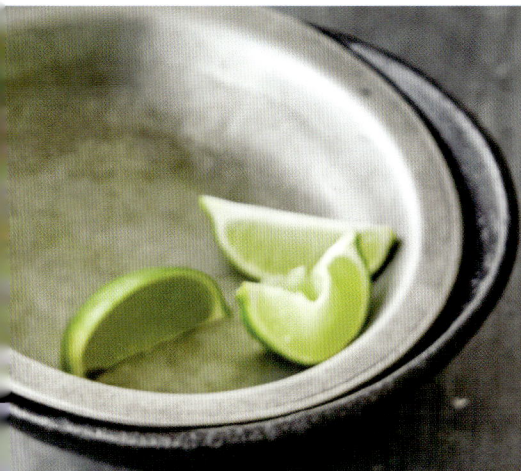

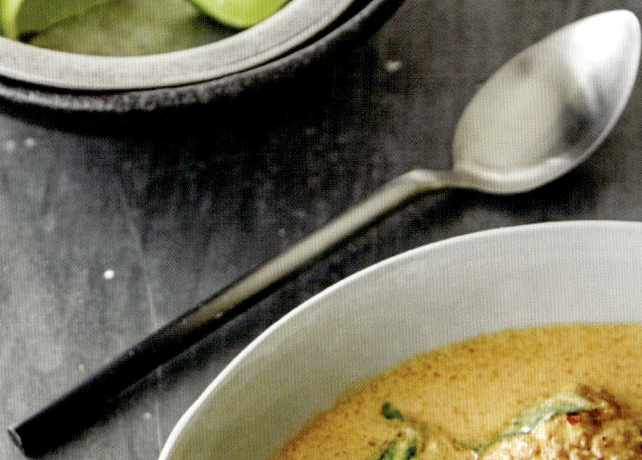

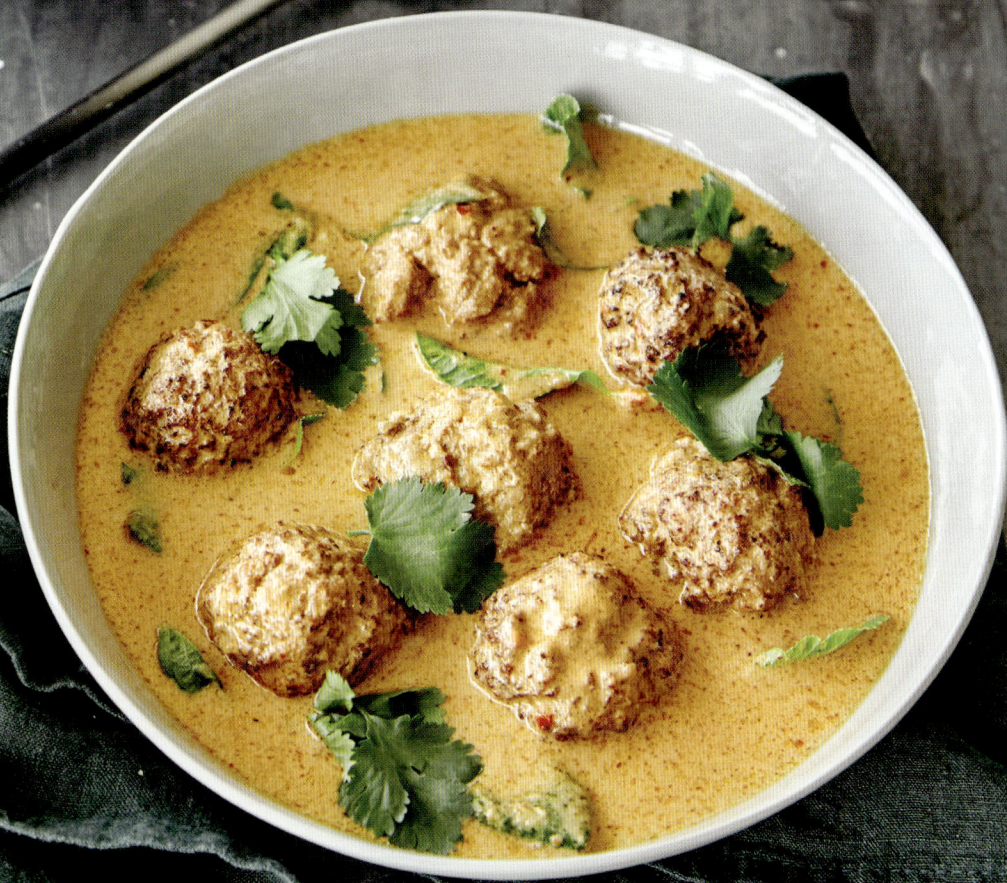

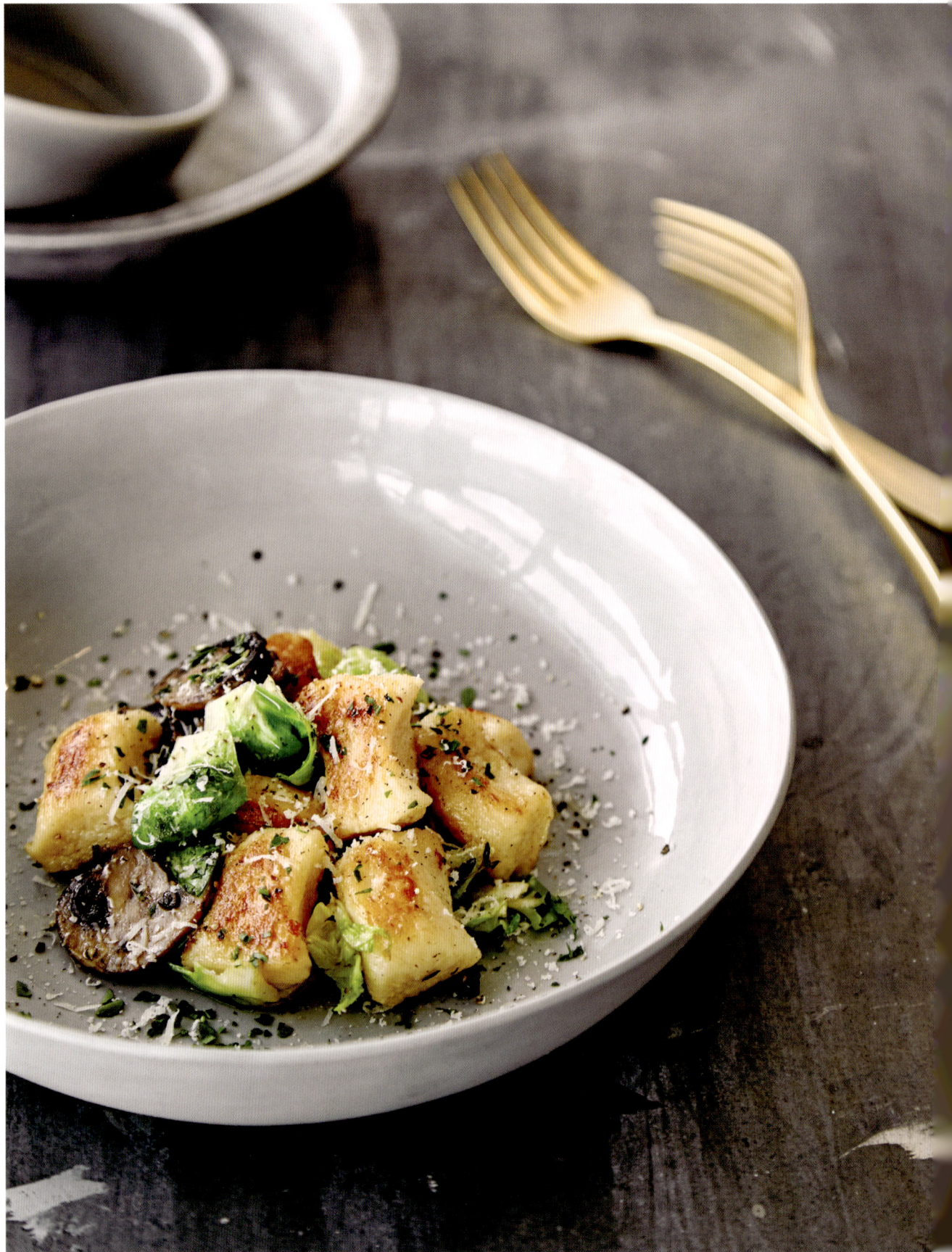

There is nothing quite as delicious as gnocchi but these temperamental dumplings can be hard to get right. When they're done wrong they can become dense and rubbery and are better suited for bouncing off a wall, however, when they are done right, they have a sublime texture that is soft yet resistant. This gnocchi is served with Brussels sprouts, mushrooms and thyme but feel free to come up with your own combinations—baby asparagus, peas and broad beans are also great when in season. For best results, this recipe requires a bag of rock salt, a potato ricer or a fine mesh sieve and, for those of you with delicate hands, a pair of disposable rubber gloves.

FRIED GNOCCHI WITH BRUSSELS SPROUTS, MUSHROOMS & THYME

Serves 6
Cooking Time: 1 hour 45 minutes

INGREDIENTS

GNOCCHI
- × 1 kg (2 lb 4 oz) desiree potatoes, unpeeled
- × 300 g (10½ oz) plain (all-purpose) flour, plus extra for dusting
- × 1 teaspoon salt
- × 2 eggs

- × 100 g (3½ oz) Brussels sprouts, leaves removed

- × 300 g (10½ oz) mushrooms, chopped
- × 2 thyme sprigs, chopped
- × 3 tablespoons olive oil
- × 3 tablespoons salt-reduced butter
- × sea salt and cracked black pepper, to season
- × 2 tablespoons continental parsley, chopped
- × parmesan cheese, grated

METHOD

Preheat the oven to 100°C (200°F/Gas 1/2).

Place the potatoes (skins on) in a pot and cover with cold water. Bring the water to a boil and then reduce to a simmer and cook for 40 minutes, or until potatoes are soft.

Spread the rock salt over a baking tray and place the potatoes on the salt, cooking them in the oven for 20 minutes. Remove the potatoes from the oven (if you need to, put on your gloves as this next part can smart a bit).

(continued)

FRIED GNOCCHI WITH BRUSSELS SPROUTS, MUSHROOMS & THYME CONTINUED...

While the potatoes are hot, press them through the ricer into a large bowl. Add the flour and salt to the potatoes. Make a well in the flour and add the eggs. Mix the ingredients until it forms a rough dough (don't overdo this part or they will be rubbery).

Dust the kitchen bench with some flour and grab a handful of dough, rolling it gently on the floured work surface into a long cigar shape.

Grab a knife and cut the dough into small sections 2 cm (¾ inches) long and place aside on a floured baking tray. Repeat until the dough is all used.

Bring pot of salted water to the boil. Remove leaves from the Brussels sprouts. Blanche the Brussels sprouts in the boiling water for 30 seconds and set aside.

Drizzle some olive oil in a non-stick pan and place over medium heat. Add the mushrooms and thyme to the pan and cook until browned on both sides. Set aside.

Add the gnocchi to a pot of boiling water and cook until they all float to the surface (this should take anywhere from 2–5 minutes).

Heat the olive oil and butter in a non-stick pan over medium heat until the butter bubbles and froths, then add the gnocchi. Cook the gnocchi on one side until golden brown, then flip and repeat.

Add the mushrooms, Brussels sprouts, then season to taste with sea salt and cracked pepper.

To serve, spoon a generous portion of gnocchi into each bowl and garnish with parsley and grated parmesan cheese. Serve with one of the simple salads (see page 103-106).

Risotto is one of those great comfort dishes that's really easy to make, delicious to eat and can be made with an almost endless variety of ingredients. The best bit about making risotto is if you are feeling like a bit of a treat the next day, you can make arancini with the leftovers. Simply roll the leftover risotto into balls with some mozzarella in the centre then coat with breadcrumbs and shallow-fry in some oil until golden.

MUSHROOM & THYME RISOTTO

Serves 4
Cooking Time: 1 hour

INGREDIENTS

× 1.25 litres (44 fl oz) chicken stock (see Basics, page 31 or unsalted if using store-bought)
× 2 tablespoons olive oil
× 500 g (1 lb 2 oz) mushrooms, thinly sliced
× 5 thyme sprigs, leaves roughly chopped
× 1 teaspoon sea salt, plus extra for serving
× 1 teaspoon cracked black pepper, plus extra for serving

× ¾ onion, diced
× 2 garlic cloves, crushed
× 300 g (10½ oz) arborio rice
× 2 tablespoons white wine vinegar
× 30 g unsalted butter
× 50 g (13/4 oz) grated parmesan cheese, plus extra for serving
× flat-leaf (Italian) parsley, finely chopped, to garnish

METHOD

Heat the chicken stock into a saucepan over low heat. Cover and leave to simmer.

Heat 1 tablespoon olive oil in a large non-stick frying pan over medium heat. When hot, add the mushrooms and thyme and season with the salt and the cracked black pepper. Cook until the mushrooms are browned. Then carefully add the mushroom mixture to the hot stock. Cover the stock and simmer for 15 minutes.

Heat the remaining olive oil in a large frying pan over low heat and add the onions and garlic. Sweat the onions, stirring constantly, until they are soft but have not coloured.

Add the rice and continue to stir, cooking until the edges of the grains have become translucent. Add the white wine vinegar and cook until the liquid is absorbed.

Increase the heat to medium and using a ladle, add the hot stock to the pan, one measure at a time, ensuring the rice is being constantly stirred as it absorbs the liquid.

(continued ↘)

MUSHROOM & THYME RISOTTO CONTINUED...

Continue to add stock and stir until most of the liquid has been used, testing the rice to ensure it has not been overcooked but the texture of the risotto is still fairly fluid (the risotto should spread across the plate when it is served).

When the rice is cooked, remove from the heat and add the butter, stirring vigorously until combined. Stir through parmesan cheese. Garnish with parsley, cracked black pepper and more parmesan cheese. Serve with one of the simple salads (page 103-106).

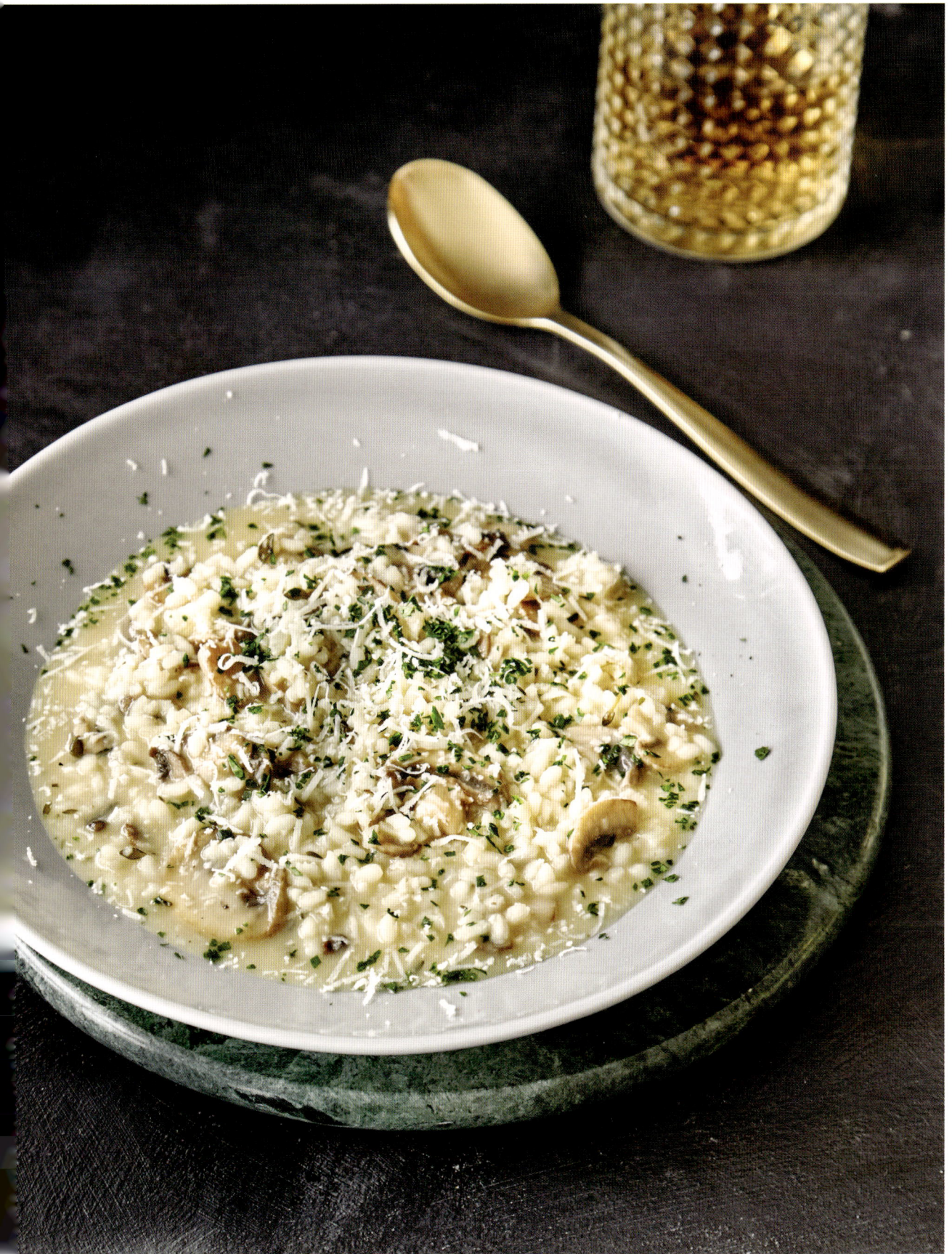

As an avid carnivore I believe it is the mark of great meal when you don't notice that it's vegetarian. This dish is packed with goodness from the spinach, chickpeas and lentils and to make it a little healthier I have also substituted the ghee with vegetable oil. If you want to take a few shortcuts, use store-bought chapati and a scoop of plain yoghurt instead of the raita.

CHICKPEA & SPINACH DHAL

Serves 6
Cooking Time: 2 hours 30 minutes

INGREDIENTS

DHAL
- × 400 g (14 oz) tinned lentils
- × 400 g (14 oz) tinned chickpeas
- × ¼ teaspoon turmeric powder
- × 750 ml (26 fl oz) chicken stock (see Basics, page 31 or unsalted if using store-bought)
- × 2 tablespoons vegetable oil
- × ¾ teaspoons coriander seeds
- × 4 garlic cloves, crushed
- × 25 g (1 oz) fresh ginger, julienned
- × 1 long green chilli, finely sliced
- × 1 red onion, finely chopped
- × 2 tomatoes, finely diced
- × 1 teaspoon garam masala powder
- × 1 teaspoon cumin
- × 80 g (23/4 oz) spinach, roughly chopped
- × ¼ bunch coriander (cilantro), roughly chopped
- × sea salt and cracked black pepper, to season

RAITA
- × 1 Lebanese (short) cucumber, grated
- × ¼ bunch coriander (cilantro), roughly chopped
- × 300 ml (101/2 fl oz) yoghurt
- × ½ teaspoons cumin
- × 1 teaspoon sea salt

CHAPATI
- × 250 g (9 oz) atta flour, plus extra for dusting
- × 1 teaspoon sea salt
- × 150 ml (5 fl oz) water

To make the Chapati dough, pour the atta flour into a mixing bowl, add the salt and make a well in the top. Slowly pour in the water a little at a time while stirring the mixture with wooden spoon until it forms a rough dough. Dust a clean work surface with flour and turn out the dough kneading for 8–10 minutes. The dough should be elastic and have a sheen to it. Coat a mixing bowl with vegetable oil and add the dough, rolling it around before covering with a tea towel and allowing to rest for at least 30 minutes.

To make the dhal, place a saucepan over medium heat and add in the lentils, chickpeas and turmeric, cover with chicken stock and bring to boil. Reduce the heat to a simmer and cook the dhal for 1 hour. Transfer to a bowl and rinse out the saucepan, then place it back over medium heat. Add the vegetable oil and when hot, add the coriander seeds and cook until they start to pop. Add the garlic, ginger and the chilli and cook until fragrant. Add the onion and half the tomato and cook for another minute, stirring frequently. Add the garam masala powder and the cumin powder. Carefully pour the dhal over the hot mixture in the saucepan and cover until it stops spitting. Uncover and reduce to a simmer, cooking for a further 10 minutes or so (the Dal should be thick when done).

To make the raita, add the cucumber, coriander and yoghurt to a bowl and season with cumin and sea salt. Mix together well and transfer to an airtight container, setting aside in the fridge.

Turn the dough out on a lightly floured work surface and cut it into six even pieces. Press each piece of dough into a roundish disc and one at a time roll out into desired shape, placing the pin across one side and quarter turning after several rolls. Place each finished piece beneath a sheet of baking paper and continue until dough is all rolled out.

Heat a cast iron skillet over medium heat until it is very hot (If you don't have a cast iron skillet you can use a normal pan) and drizzle some vegetable oil and place dough in the pan.

Cook the chapati until they are mottled and delicious on both sides, then remove from the heat and set aside under a tea towel to keep warm. Repeat this process with all of the dough.

Season the dhal with salt and pepper and stir in the spinach, coriander and the remaining tomatoes. Serve over brown rice with chapatis and a tablespoon of raita over the top.

Here are some super simple pastas that taste great and are an easy option for dinner, especially if you're looking for something quick to whip up when you get home from work. All of these recipes go great with dried pasta but if you have the time, trying making the fettuccine from scratch, you will be amazed by the difference.

FETTUCCINE WITH A SPINACH, MUSHROOM AND WALNUT PESTO

Serves 4
Cooking Time: 30 minutes

INGREDIENTS

- × 200g (7 oz) mushrooms, chopped
- × 80g (3 oz) walnuts
- × 100g (3 ½ oz) baby spinach leaves
- × 1 clove of garlic, peeled

- × 50g (2 oz) parmesan cheese, grated plus extra for garnish
- × 50ml (3 ½ fl oz) olive oil, plus extra for frying
- × 400g (15 oz) fettuccine
- × sea salt and cracked black pepper, to season

METHOD

Fill a pot with water, add some salt and bring to a rolling boil (water should be a salty as the Mediterranean, not the Dead Sea).

Heat some olive oil in a non-stick frying pan over medium heat. Add the mushrooms, cooking until slightly browned. Remove from heat.

Grab a food processor and add the mushrooms, walnuts, baby spinach, garlic and parmesan. Blitz until there are no big chunks, then with the motor running add the olive oil in a thin steady stream until the oil is incorporated.

Cook pasta until *al dente* and drain (save a couple of tablespoons of the starchy pasta water).

Heat a drizzle of olive oil in a non-stick frying pan over medium heat and add the pesto. Add the pasta water to the pesto to loosen it up then and pasta. Toss together well and season with sea salt and cracked black pepper then remove from heat.

Serve while hot with a generous amount of parmesan cheese and a Simple Salad (page 103-106).

PENNE WITH BROAD BEANS, BABY ASPARAGUS AND PEAS.

Serves 4
Cooking Time: 30 minutes

INGREDIENTS

- × 100g (3 ½ oz) baby asparagus, roughly chopped
- × 100g (3 ½ oz) broad beans, shelled
- × 100g (3 ½ oz) peas
- × 1 clove of garlic, peeled and finely chopped
- × 3 tablespoons of olive oil

- × 20g (1 oz) unsalted butter
- × 400g (15 oz) penne
- × sea salt and cracked black pepper, to season
- × 40g (1 ½ oz) parmesan cheese, grated

METHOD

Fill a pot with water, add some salt and bring to a rolling boil (water should be a salty as the Mediterranean, not the Dead Sea).

Add the baby asparagus, broad beans and peas to the water and cook for a minute, fish them out with a slotted spoon and place them in a strainer. Run them under a could tap for a few seconds to refresh and put aside.

Cook pasta until *al dente* and drain (save a couple of tablespoons of the starchy pasta water).

Heat the olive oil and butter in a non-stick frying pan over medium heat. Add the garlic, cooking until slightly coloured then the baby asparagus, broad beans and peas. Add the pasta and pasta water then toss together, seasoning with sea salt and cracked black pepper then remove from heat.

Serve while hot with a generous amount of parmesan cheese and a Simple Salad (page 103-106).

RIGATONI WITH TUNA AND BLACK OLIVES

Serves 4
Cooking Time: 30 minutes

INGREDIENTS

- × 2 x 400g (15 oz) cans whole peeled tomatoes
- × 2 tablespoons olive oil, plus extra for frying
- × 2 cloves of garlic, peeled and finely diced
- × 500g (16 oz) tuna fillet, chopped roughly
- × 100g (3 ½ oz) black olives, pitted and roughly chopped

- × 1 teaspoon of dried chilli flakes (optional)
- × 400g (15 oz) rigatoni
- × ¼ bunch continental parsley, roughly chopped
- × ½ lemon, juiced
- × sea salt and cracked black pepper, to season

MTHOD

Fill a pot with water, add some salt and bring to a rolling boil (water should be a salty as the Mediterranean, not the Dead Sea).

Place the tomatoes into a bowl and break them up roughly with a potato masher.

Heat some olive oil in a non-stick frying pan over medium heat. Add the garlic cloves, cooking until slightly coloured, then add the tomatoes, the tuna, black olives and chilli flakes (optional). Bring to boil then drop to a simmer for 15 minutes.

Cook pasta until *al dente*, drain (save a couple of tablespoons of the starchy pasta water).

Use a fork to break apart the tuna chunks, add the pasta water then season with sea salt and cracked black pepper. Add the pasta to the pan, toss together well then remove from heat.

Place the pasta in a large serving bowl and top with the continental parsley, lemon juice, 2 tablespoons of olive oil and a couple of extra cracks of black pepper.

Serve while hot with a Simple Salad (page 103-106).

CRAVINGS

From The Wife

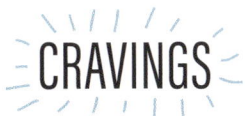

So, as far as cravings go this dish should be at the top of the list: a traditional, old school lasagne with an Osso Bucco & Pork Shoulder Ragù. Compared to some other lasagne recipes this one does take a little more time but let me tell you, it is most definitely worth the effort and a great thing to make on a lazy Sunday afternoon. The problem with this dish is once you taste the combination of the rich ragù with the creamy béchamel and gooey mozzarella, you will become hooked.

OSSO BUCCO & PORK SHOULDER LASAGNE

Serves 6

Cooking Time: 4 hours and 30 minutes

INGREDIENTS

OSSO BUCCO & PORK SHOULDER RAGÙ

- × 1 oregano sprig
- × 1 rosemary sprig
- × 1 thyme sprig
- × 1 continental parsley sprig
- × 500 g (1 lb 2 oz) osso bucco
- × 500 g (1 lb 2 oz) pork shoulder, chopped into chunks
- × 1 tablespoon sea salt
- × 1 tablespoon cracked black pepper
- × 2 tablespoons olive oil
- × 1 onion, roughly chopped
- × 10 garlic cloves
- × 3 tablespoons red wine vinegar
- × 800 g (1 lb 12 oz) tinned whole peeled tomatoes

- × 1 litre (35 fl oz) beef stock (see Basics, page 32 or unsalted if using store bought)

BÉCHAMEL SAUCE
(Makes 800 ml/28 fl oz)
- × 65 g (21/4 oz) butter
- × 40 g (1½ oz) plain (all-purpose) flour
- × pinch of nutmeg
- × 600 ml (21 fl oz) milk
- × 1 bay leaf

- × 1 box lasagne sheets
- × 300 g (10 oz) mozzarella cheese, grated
- × 60 g (6 oz) parmesan cheese, grated
- × ½ bunch continental parsley, roughly chopped

Continued ⌐

MORE SUBSTANTIAL

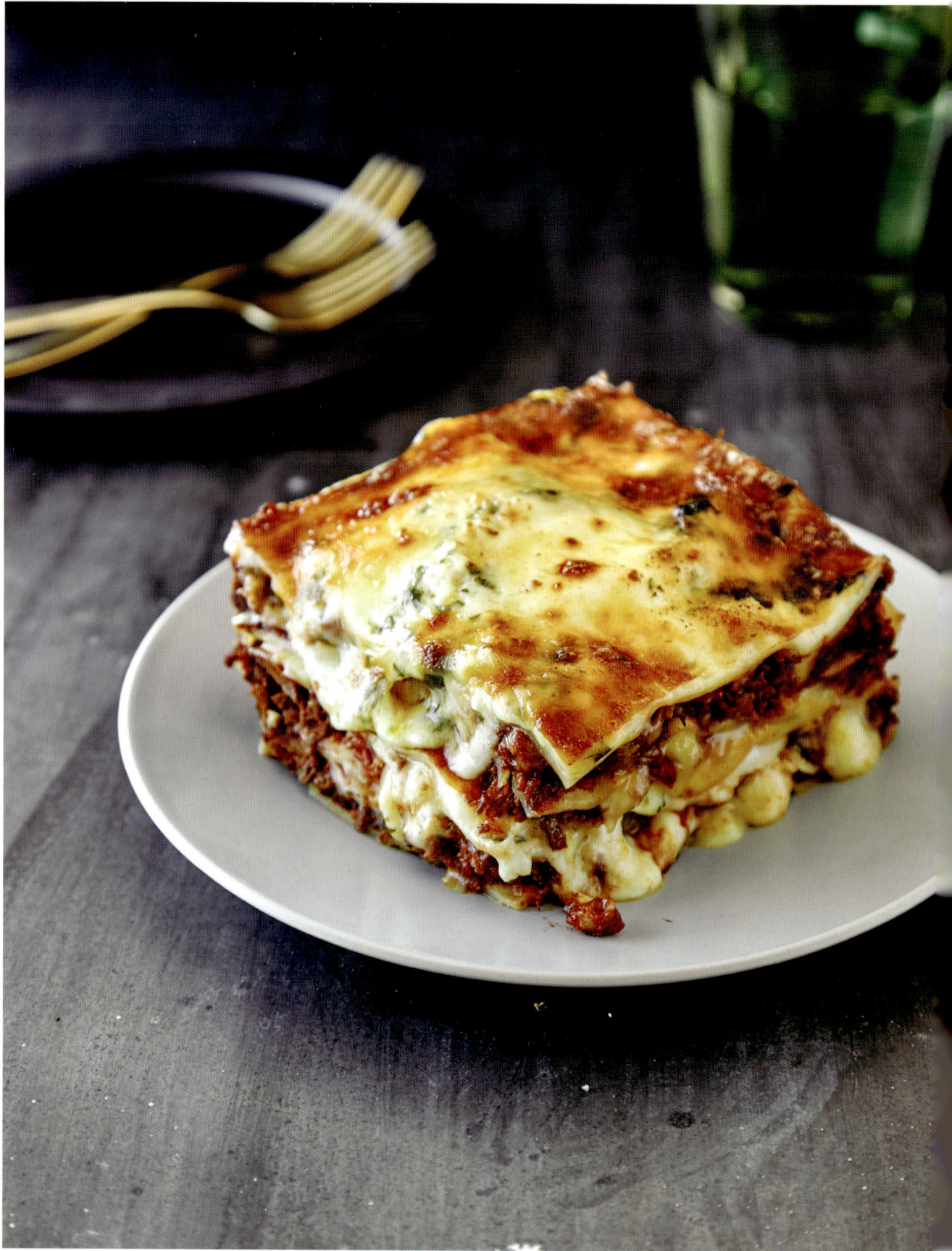

OSSO BUCCO & PORK SHOULDER LASAGNE CONTINUED...

Gather the oregano, rosemary, thyme and continental parsley and tie together securely with a length of kitchen string to make a bouquet garni.

Season the osso bucco and pork shoulder with the sea salt and cracked black pepper. Place a large pot over medium heat and add the olive oil. When hot, add the osso bucco and pork shoulder, browning on all sides. Add the onion and the garlic. Add the red wine vinegar and scrape all of the brown from the bottom of the pot. Add the tomatoes and beef stock and stir well. Cover, bring to the boil and then reduce to a low simmer. Cook for 2 hours. Remove the lid and reduce for a further 30 minutes, stirring frequently. (You will know when dish is cooked because the meat will be tender and fall apart.) Pick out the bouquet garni, bones and any fat from the osso bucco and break up all the meat with a wooden spoon

To make the béchamel sauce, place a saucepan over low heat and add the butter. When the butter is melted, add the flour and nutmeg stirring to combine well. Continue stirring while pouring the milk into the saucepan in a thin stream until it is all combined. Add the bay leaf and simmer until the béchamel has thickened. Remove the bay leaf and set aside in the fridge.

Preheat the oven to 180°C (350°F) and grease an ovenproof dish with olive oil. Lay a layer of lasagne sheets on the bottom of the dish. Spoon over the ragù and top with béchamel. Add a layer of mozzarella cheese, parmesan cheese and continental parsley. Top with a layer of lasagne sheets and repeat the layers finishing the dish with a top layer of béchamel and mozzarella. Place into the oven and cook for 40 minutes. Remove and leave to stand for 15 minutes before serving. Serve with one of the simple salads (see page 103-106).

MORE SUBSTANTIAL

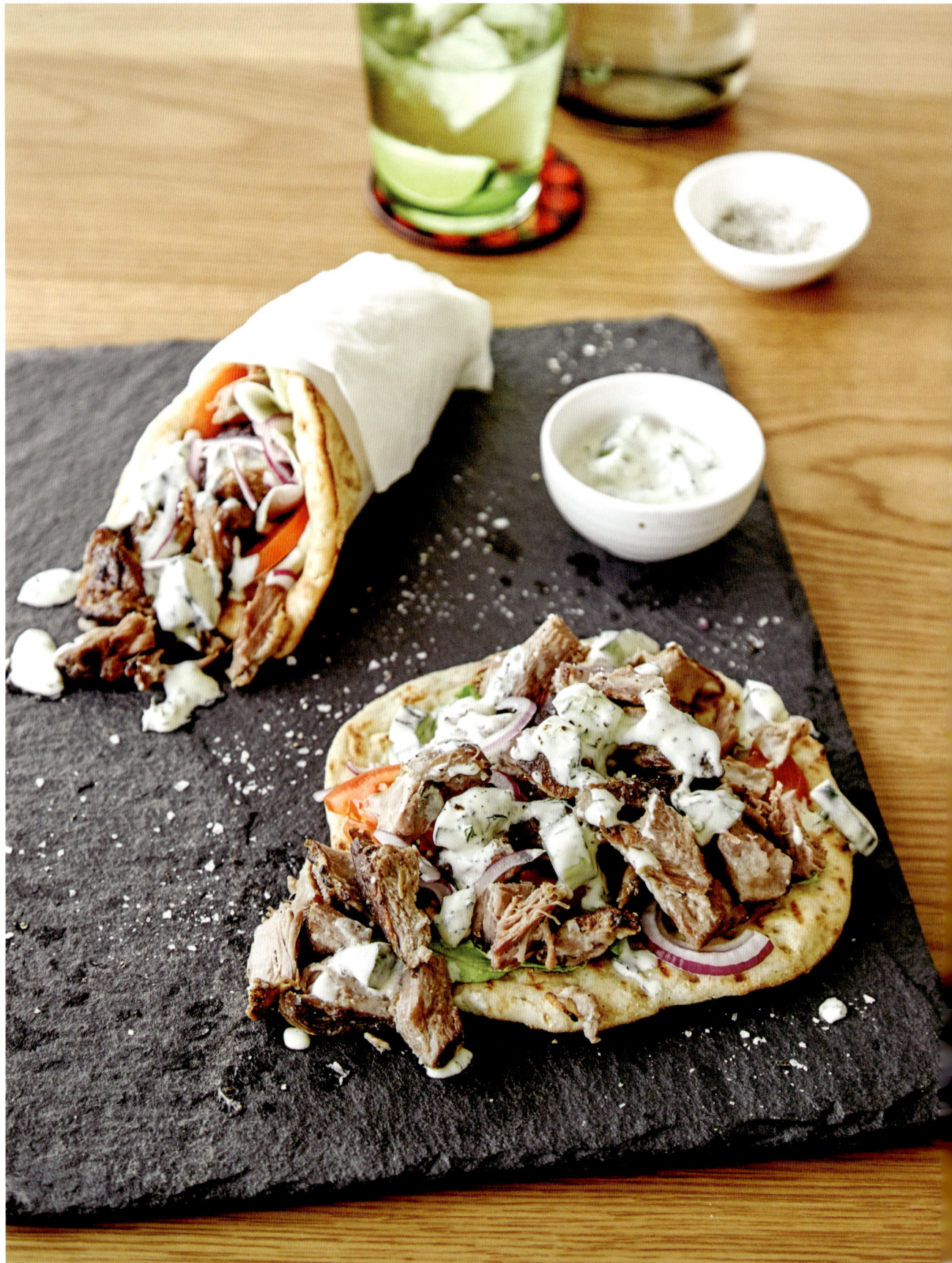

One of the hard things about getting takeout for an expectant mother is the limitations on what they can and cannot eat. So one of the easiest way around this is to make it yourself. Now this recipe calls for you to make the roast lamb, tzatziki and the pita bread. If you are time poor by all means just do the meat but if you have the time one Sunday afternoon make the whole recipe, you will not regret it. I promise.

ROAST LAMB SOUVLAKI

Serves 6
Cooking Time: 2 hours 50 minutes

INGREDIENTS

PITA BREAD
(If you are going to use store-bought make sure you heat them in a pan for a few seconds per side before serving)
× 1 sachet instant yeast powder
× 1 teaspoon sugar
× 410 g (14½ oz) plain (all-purpose) flour, plus extra for dusting
× 2 teaspoons salt
× 3 tablespoons olive oil

ROAST LAMB
× 1.4 kg (3 lb) half lamb leg
× 3 garlic cloves, quartered
× 3 sprigs rosemary, roughly torn
× 1 tablespoon olive oil
× juice of half a lemon
× 1 tablespoon sea salt

× ½ red onion, thinly sliced
× 2 tomatoes, thinly sliced
× ¼ iceberg lettuce
× 6 tablespoons Tzatziki (see Basics, page 37 or store bought)

METHOD

To make the pita bread, place 1 sachet of instant yeast powder in a mixing bowl and add 250 ml (9 fl oz) warm water. Mix together and cover for 10 minutes. If it bubbles, the yeast is active if not, discard and start again. Add the sugar, flour, salt and olive oil to the bowl and combine until you have a rough dough.

Dust a clean work surface with flour and turn out the dough, kneading for 8–10 minutes. The dough should be elastic and have a sheen to it.

Coat a mixing bowl in olive oil and add the dough, rubbing the exterior in olive oil before covering with a tea towel and allowing to rise for at least 2 hours.

Continued ⤷

ROAST LAMB SOUVLAKI CONTINUED...

Preheat the oven to 180°C (350°F/Gas 4). Place the lamb in a roasting tray and cut 12 deep incisions across the surface, stuffing the holes with a piece of garlic and rosemary. Drizzle the lamb with olive oil and lemon juice and season with sea salt. Place lamb in the oven and roast for 1 hour.

Remove the tray from the oven and using tongs, carefully turn the lamb over, returning to the oven for a further 45 minutes. Remove the lamb from oven and rest for 15 minutes.

To finish the pita bread, the dough should have finished rising so punch it back down into a ball and turn in out on a lightly floured work surface. Cut it into six even pieces. Press each piece of dough into a roundish disc and one at a time roll out into desired shape, placing the pin across one side and quarter turning after several rolls. Place each finished piece beneath a sheet of baking paper and continue until dough is all rolled out.

Heat a cast iron skillet over medium heat until it is very hot. Brush one side of the bread with olive oil a place oil side down in the pan. While the first side is cooking brush the other side with olive oil and flip when mottled brown and blackened. Repeat this process with all of the flat breads and wrap in foil to keep nice and warm.

Cut the lamb into thin slices, removing the bone, then using two forks pull apart the meat into shreds, covering with the pan juices.

Lay pita bread on a plate, slather with tzatziki and add a generous amount of lamb and top with onions. Add the tomato and lettuce, then roll up and serve.

NEW USES FOR OLD BABY STUFF

The reality of being a new parent really sinks in the first time you walk into one of those enormous baby emporiums that seem to stretch off towards some distant horizon, every square centimetre of the floor space crammed with aisle after aisle of strange and colourful products you have never seen nor heard of before. And as you stand at the door of these maternal merchandising meccas trying to figure out what to do and where to start, the horrible truth dawns on you that you will probably need to own at least one of every item that they have in stock.

Breast pumps, baby baths, bassinets, baby blenders, bath seats, baby walkers, bibs, booster seats, bottles, bottle warmers, bottle brushes, baby swings, baby monitors the list is ten miles long and that's just some of the Bs. Throw in daycare and you suddenly find your wallet is haemorrhaging money so badly that you'll start getting calls from salivating credit card companies offering to up your limit as they circle slowly above your soon to be bankrupt corpse like vultures.

And we haven't even considered paying for schooling yet.

What is even harder is knowing that most of the stuff you spend your hard earned dollars on will be redundant within the first couple of years and you will be grinning through gritted teeth as you hand over those hardly used, very expensive items to the friends or family that were smart enough to have a baby nine months after you. So to compensate I have come up with a few alternate uses for some everyday baby items.

The first time you bathe your newborn child in their very own little baby tub is a touching and wonderful moment that you will always remember. But did you know that baby baths also make excellent drinks coolers? Your partner will adore your sentimentality when you pack that little tub of memories full of ice, wine and beer at your next barbecue or dinner party, and the best bit is, most of them come with plugs for easy drainage!

Prams don't come cheap; in fact, they can be one of the most expensive baby items you buy. But did you know they are also great for hauling groceries and other cumbersome items? Simply lay the seat flat, stack the pram full of shopping and make the little one walk. Sure, you may get some strange looks from people you pass in the street but as long as you remember to take the child out before you load it up there shouldn't be a problem at all.

But it doesn't end there, there is a use for everything once your baby outgrows them. Swaddles are great for polishing the car, portable bottle warmers keep your coffee piping hot on the way to work, baby monitors make great security cameras, bibs can be repurposed for adults to wear at your next barbecue.

But if you really want to save some money my advice would be to have a little foresight and make sure you carefully unwrap and save the packaging from the millions of wraps, sleeping bags, swaddles and toys you have over bought or have been given doubles of since the birth. Because as long as the stains wash out, nobody will be any the wiser when you cleverly re-gift them at the next baby shower you've been invited to.

That includes this book too!

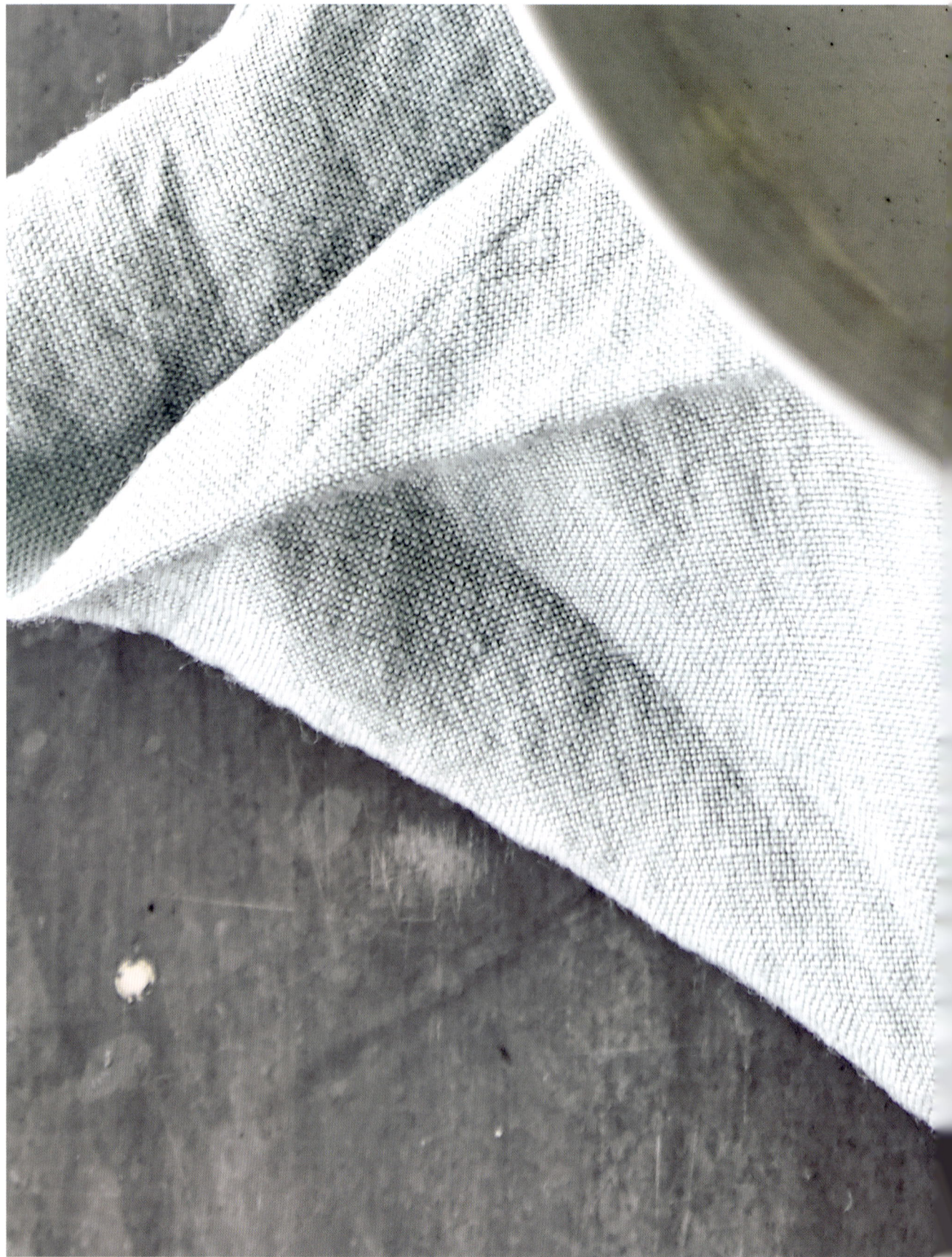

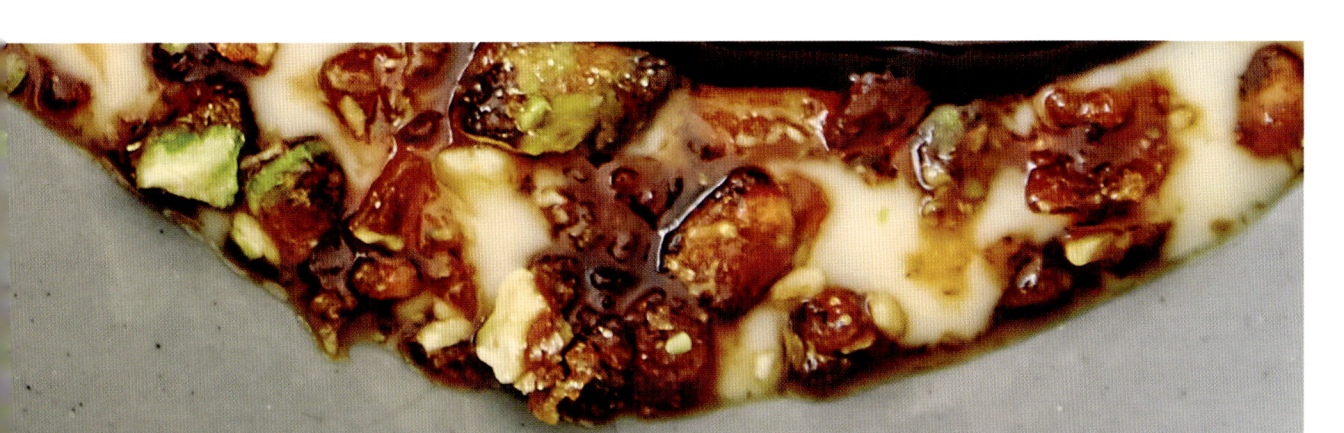

SOMETHING SWEET

Some treats that are actually good for you (and quite a few that aren't).

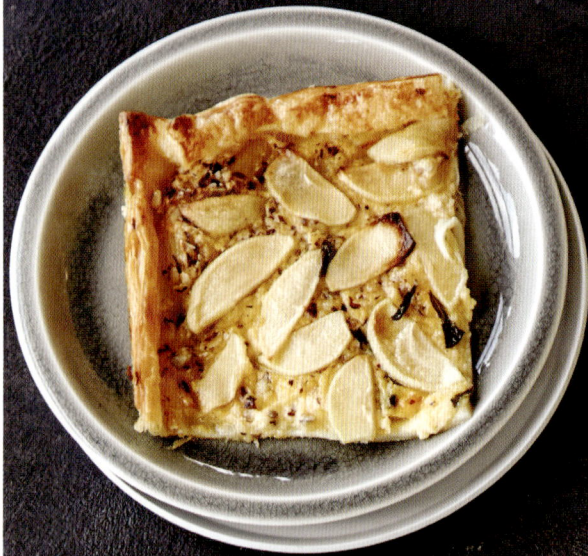

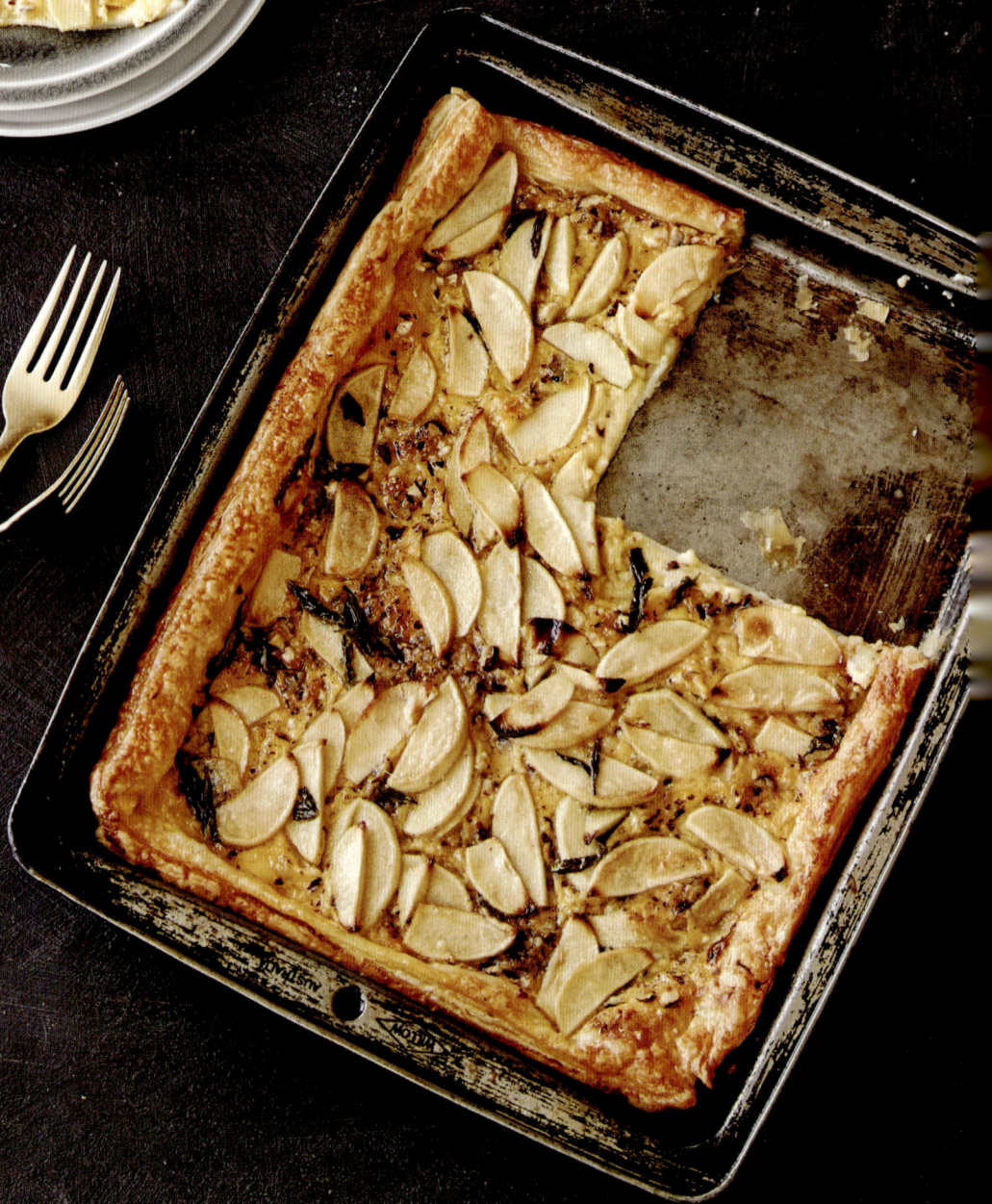

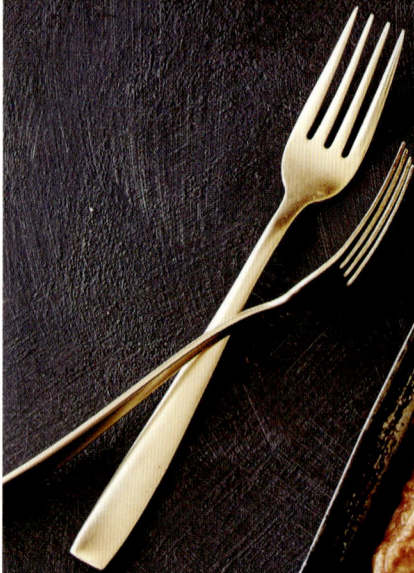

This recipe is one of my favourites because you don't have to make pastry (which is great because I'm not that good at it). Although the tart is baked I have substituted the eggs normally found in the pastry cream for cornflour to be on the safe side. This dish uses apples and tarragon but these can easily be substituted for pears, peaches or cherries.

APPLE, HAZELNUT & TARRAGON TART

Serves 6
Cooking Time: 1 hour 15 minutes

INGREDIENTS

- × 1 tablespoon unsalted butter
- × 2½ tablespoons honey
- × 25 g (1 oz) hazelnuts
- × 300 ml (10½ fl oz) milk
- × 1 cinnamon quill
- × 5 tarragon sprigs, roughly chopped

- × 2 teaspoons vanilla extract
- × 3 green apples, peeled, quartered and thinly sliced
- × 100 ml (3½ fl oz) thick cream
- × 50 g (1¾ oz) caster (superfine) sugar
- × 10 g (½ oz) cornflour (cornstarch)
- × 1 sheet of puff pastry (enough to line a baking tray)

METHOD

Preheat the oven to 180°C (350°F/Gas 4) and grease a baking tray.

Place the butter and 1 tablespoon of the honey in a saucepan over medium heat and melt. Set aside for later.

Using a mortar and pestle, food processor or a tea towel and a rolling pin, crush the hazelnuts so they are roughly broken up.

Place a dry frying pan over medium heat and toast the hazelnuts until fragrant. Set aside in a bowl.

Place a saucepan over medium heat and add the milk, cinnamon, chopped tarragon and vanilla extract. Bring the milk to the boil and then reduce to a simmer for 5 minutes. Stand for a further 5 minutes.

Add the apple to a mixing bowl. Sprinkle the remaining tarragon sprigs over the apples. Drizzle over the honey and toss together well and set aside.

Add the cream, caster sugar and cornflour to a bowl and whisk together so there are no lumps. Grab a fine mesh sieve and pour the milk mixture through and into the bowl with the cream and whisk together. Pour the mixture into a clean saucepan and return to low heat. Cook and stir the mixture until it is a thick custard, then remove from the heat and stand for 5 minutes.

Continued

APPLE, HAZELNUT & TARRAGON TART CONTINUED...

Place the puff pastry on the baking tray, pressing firmly around the edges and then prick it with a fork. Grab a pastry brush and apply a liberal coating of the melted butter and honey mixture to the pastry (make sure about half is left). Coat the pastry in a thick layer of the tarragon-infused pastry cream and then sprinkle the toasted hazelnuts over the top.

Place the apples over the surface of the tart and press them into the cream, then glaze with the remainder of the melted butter and honey mixture.

Bake for 30 minutes, then remove from the oven and leave to stand for 10 minutes. Serve hot with some plum & cherry frozen yoghurt (see page 194).

Funtastic Baby Facts
Newborns can take anywhere from 5 minutes to an hour to feed.

I am a sucker for pumpkin pie, although I must admit when I was younger it struck me as one of the oddest dishes in the entire world. Pumpkin pie is a wonderful combination of the dark flavors of roasted pumpkin, the sweetness of molasses and the earthiness of cinnamon, cloves, ginger and nutmeg in one delicious mouthful. However, it takes a long time to make it right. So here are some tips if you want to cut down the cooking time. Number one: Steam the pumpkin instead of roasting. Two: Use store-bought pastry. Three: Don't blind bake the crust first. Skipping these steps will cut about 1 hour out of the cooking time, you may not get the same result but you will have more time to help around the house!

PUMPKIN & PECAN PIE

Serves 6
Cooking Time: 2 hours 15 minutes

INGREDIENTS

PASTRY OR 1 SHEET OF STORE BOUGHT SHORTCRUST PASTRY

× 250 g (9 oz) plain (all-purpose) flour
× 1 tablespoon icing (confectioners') sugar
× pinch of salt
× 125g (4½ oz) unsalted butter, chilled
× 1 egg, chilled
× 1 tablespoon water, chilled

PUMPKIN PIE FILLING

× 1 small butternut pumpkin (squash), peeled, cored and cut into small pieces.
× 110 g (33/4 oz) pecans
× 1 teaspoon dried ginger
× ½ teaspoons dried cloves
× ½ teaspoons nutmeg
× ½ teaspoons ground cinnamon
× 4 eggs
× 185 g (6½ oz) firmly packed brown sugar
× 3 tablespoons molasses
× 375 ml (13 fl oz) tinned evaporated milk

(Continued ⤵)

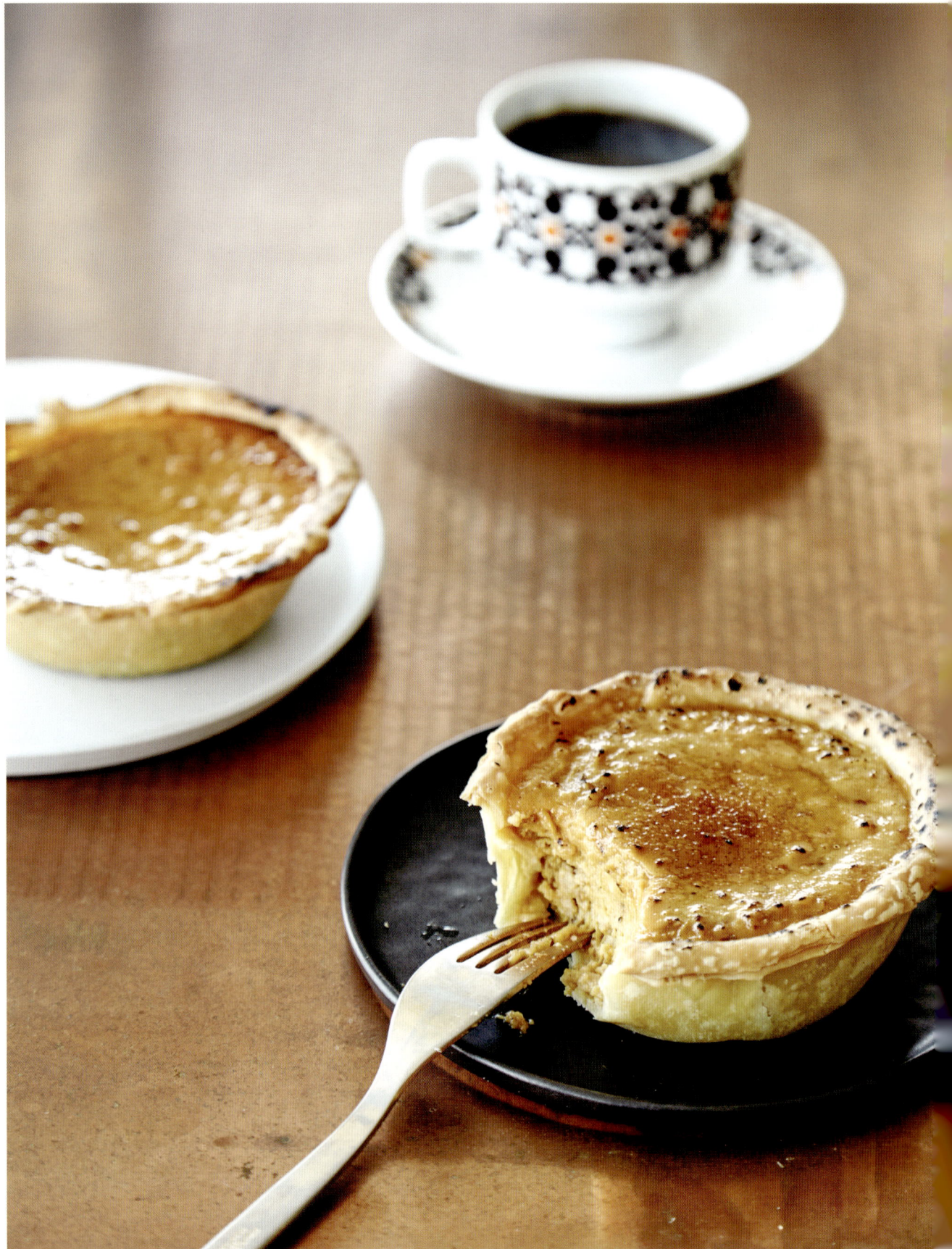

PUMPKIN & PECAN PIE CONTINUED...

Preheat the oven to 180°C (350°F/Gas 4). Place the pumpkin on a baking tray and roast for 20 minutes, or until slightly browned and blackened.

Place the pecans onto a chopping board and crush them using a rolling pin.

Place a dry frying pan over low heat, add the pecans and roast until fragrant, then set aside. Return the frying pan to the stovetop over low heat and roast the ginger, cloves, nutmeg and cinnamon until fragrant.

Place the pumpkin, ginger, cloves, nutmeg and cinnamon into a food processor and process until combined.

Place the eggs into a large mixing bowl and whisk. Add the brown sugar, pumpkin mix, molasses and evaporated milk and whisk together vigorously until combined. Add the pecans and fold through. Let sit for 1 hour covered in the fridge.

To make the pastry, chop the butter into small cubes and set aside in the fridge. Place the egg in a small bowl and whisk. Set aside in the fridge.

Clear a workspace and sieve the flour and icing sugar on your bench, then add the salt. Add the butter and work through by pinching the pieces of butter into the flour until it resembles a chunky breadcrumbs

Remove the whisked eggs from the fridge and add the chilled water, stirring until combined. Add the mixture to the flour and work with your hands until mixture begins to form large clumps. (Don't overwork the dough as the butter may melt). Bring together into a rough dough and then form into a disc. Wrap the dough in plastic wrap and refrigerate for at least 30 minutes.

Preheat the oven to 220°C (425°F/Gas 7). Grease a pie dish with some butter.

Lightly flour a clean work surface and remove the pastry from refrigerator. Using a rolling pin, roll out the pastry until it is a large disc the will easily fit into you pie dish (Remember, being too big and trimming is better than too small).

Line the pie dish with the pastry, ensuring it is pressed down in the corners and prick the bottom of the pastry gently with a fork. Place the pie dish in the fridge for 15 minutes.

Remove the pie dish from the fridge and place a sheet of baking paper in the centre of the dish and fill with uncooked rice and blind bake for 10 minutes.

Remove the paper and the rice weights and return the pie shell to the oven for a further 5 minutes. Remove the pie shell from the oven, trim away any excess edges and get the pumpkin mixture from the fridge.

Gently pour the mixture into the pie shell ensuring it is evenly distributed. Reduce the oven temperature to 170°C (325°F/Gas 3) and bake for 45 minutes, or until the filling is set. Remove pie from oven and set aside to cool.

Serve with a scoop of coconut, date & molasses frozen yoghurt (see page 196) on the side.

While this dish may bring instant connotations of big hair, ripped jeans and flashbacks to the 80s it is actually a delicious dessert that's easy to make. If cherries are out of season (or you just too lazy to pit them) feel free to use the frozen kind.

CHERRY PIE

Serves 4
Cooking Time: 1 hour

INGREDIENTS

× 150 g (5 1/2 oz) cherries
× 3 tablespoons honey
× 1 tablespoon caster (superfine) sugar
× 80 g (2¾ oz) unsalted butter

× 10 filo pastry sheets
× 50 g (1¾ oz) almond meal
× 3 tablespoons caster (superfine) sugar, plus additional for topping

METHOD

Preheat the oven to 180°C (350°F/Gas 4). Lightly grease a baking tray.

Destem and remove the cherry pits placing the flesh into a mixing bowl. Pour the honey over the cherries and add the sugar, tossing until they are mixed together well. Set aside.

Place a small saucepan over low heat and melt the butter. Brush each sheet of filo with melted butter and lay on top of each other. Place the cherry mixture in the centre of the buttered filo pastry. Sprinkle the mixture with the almond meal. Fold the ends of the filo pastry towards the centre. Fold the sides of the filo pastry over the ends until in forms a neat package and brush again with butter.

Cut three small diagonal slices across the top of the pastry and place on the baking tray, sprinkling with a little sugar. Place the baking tray into the oven and bake for 25 minutes. Remove the baking tray from the oven and rest the cherry pie for 15 minutes before serving.

Serve hot with some plum & cherry frozen yoghurt (page 194) on the side.

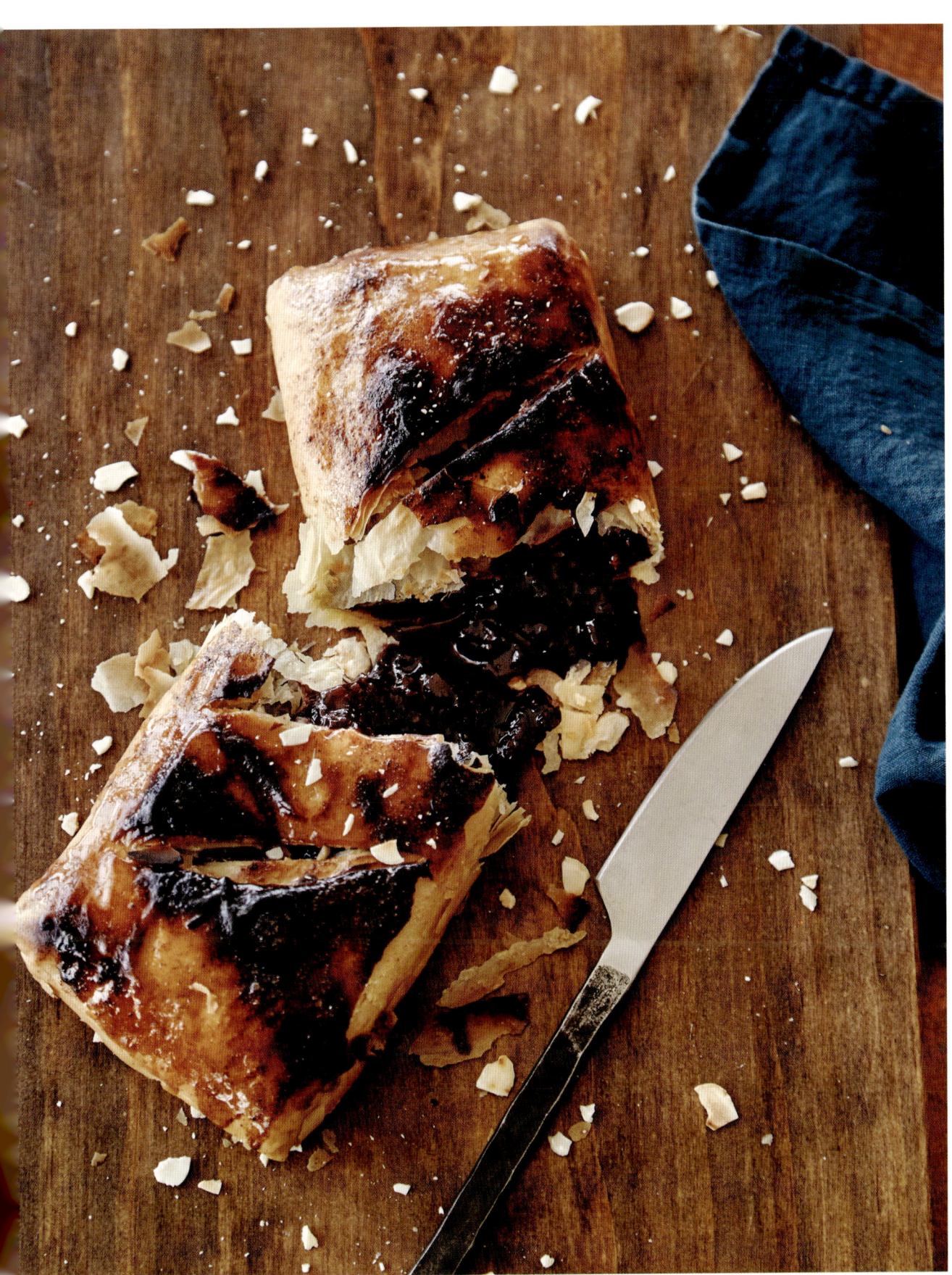

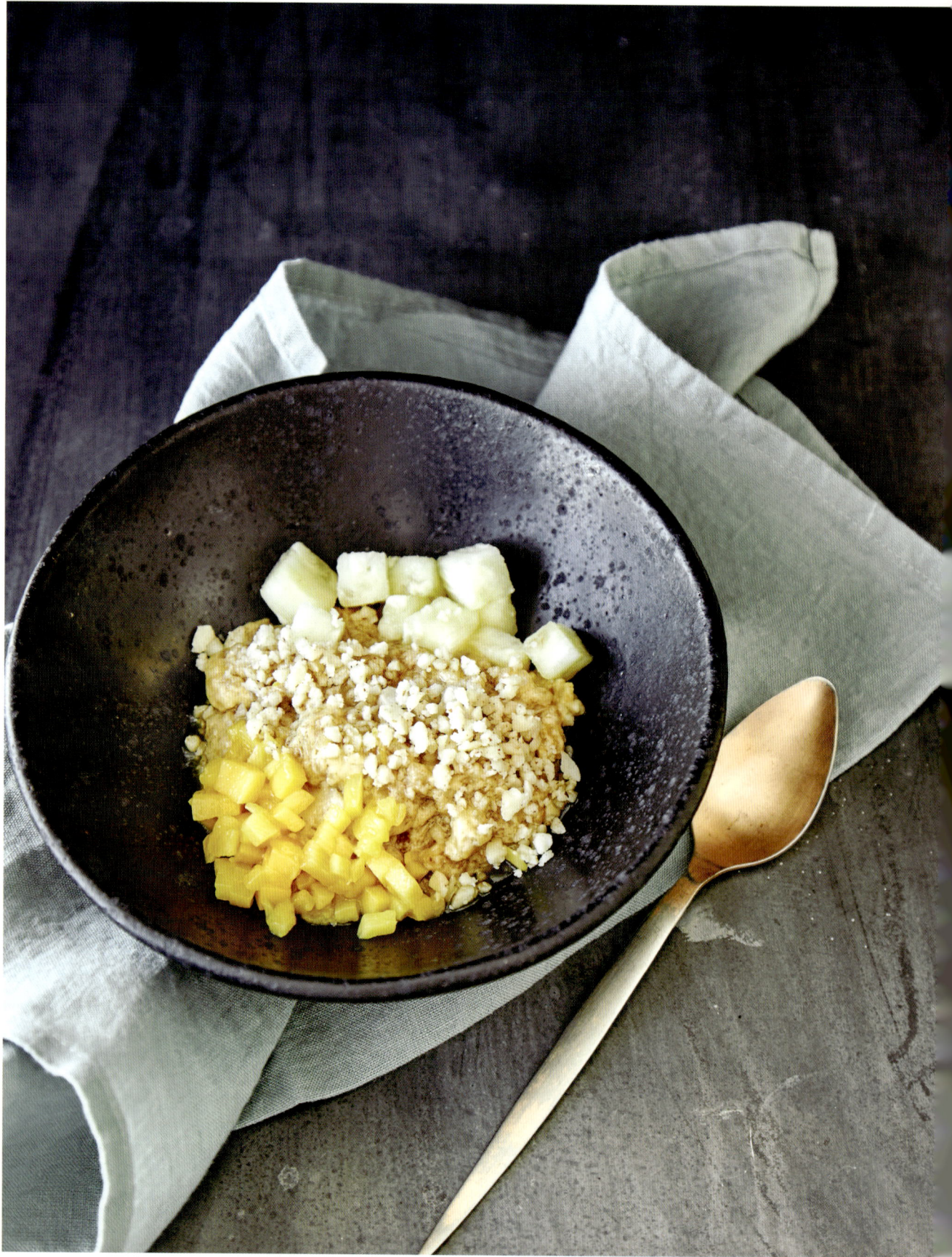

oh, how I loved rice pudding as a little kid, it was one of my favourite things that my parents made for dessert. But as we all know rice, milk and sugar probably aren't the best things in the world for an expectant mother so I have added a coconutty kind of tropical twist to the dish which makes it more like one of the sweet rice porridges you might find in South-East Asia.

PASSIONFRUIT, PINEAPPLE & COCONUT RICE PUDDING

Serves 6
Cooking Time: 1 hour 35 minutes

INGREDIENTS

× 50 g (13/4 oz) macadamia nuts
× 4 tablespoons desiccated coconut
× 750 ml (26 fl oz) tinned coconut milk
× 1 piece of lemon zest
× 1 teaspoon vanilla extract
× 2 tablespoons honey
× 2 tablespoons golden syrup
× 2 tablespoons molasses
× 140 g (5 oz) arborio rice
× 1 mango, diced
× ¼ pineapple, diced
× 2 passionfruit
× ½ lime

METHOD

Preheat the oven to 180°C (350°F/Gas 4).

Use a mortar and pestle, food processor, or a tea towel and rolling pin, crush the macadamia nuts so they are roughly broken up.

Place a dry frying pan over medium heat and toast the macadamia nuts and desiccated coconut until fragrant. Set aside in a bowl.

Add the coconut milk to a saucepan and place over low heat. Add the lemon zest, vanilla extract, honey, golden syrup and molasses. Bring the milk to the boil, then reduce to a simmer for 10 minutes. Remove from the heat and leave to stand for a further 5 minutes.

Remove the lemon and add the rice. Bring the ingredients to a boil, then carefully pour into a casserole or similar high ovenproof dish.

Continued ⤵

PASSIONFRUIT, PINEAPPLE & COCONUT RICE PUDDING CONTINUED...

Bake for 1 hour, then remove from the oven and leave to stand for 10 minutes. The rice should have absorbed the liquid (if not you can put it back in the oven for another 10 minutes if you like).

Add the mango and pineapple to a mixing bowl. Slice the passionfruit and scoop out over the top of the fruit and mix well.

To serve, add a generous amount of the rice pudding to a bowl and top with toasted macadamia nuts, desiccated coconut and mango pineapple mix.

For an extra treat you can add a scoop of blueberry & maple syrup frozen yoghurt (see page 197).

From The Wife

I will agree that fried bananas aren't that great for you. Pudding isn't the healthiest option either and let's not even started on the brittle. So you'd better limit this dish to just those nights when the temptation of crisp fried banana, creamy pudding and sweet, crunchy brittle is just too great to ignore. Just so you know, it tastes pretty good with hot chocolate fudge as well.

FRIED BANANA PUDDING WITH PISTACHIO BRITTLE

Serves 4
Cooking Time: 1 hour 30 minutes

NGREDIENTS

PISTACHIO BRITTLE
- × 120 g (41/4 oz) caster (superfine) sugar
- × 2 tablespoons water
- × 40 g (1½ oz) pistachios
- × pinch of sea salt

BANANA PUDDING
- × 300 ml (101/2 fl oz) milk
- × 200 ml (7 fl oz) thick cream
- × 1 teaspoon cinnamon
- × 1 tablespoon brown sugar
- × 3 tablespoons golden syrup

- × 1 teaspoon vanilla extract
- × 3 bananas
- × 1 tablespoon cornflour (cornstarch)

FRIED BANANA
- × 100 g (4 oz) plain (all-purpose) flour, plus extra for coating
- × pinch of salt
- × ½ teaspoons bicarbonate of soda (baking soda)
- × 170 ml (51/2 fl oz) soda water
- × 2 bananas
- × 125 ml (4 fl oz) vegetable oil

METHOD

For the pistachio brittle, use a mortar and pestle, or a tea towel and rolling pin, crush the pistachios so they are roughly broken up.
Line a tray with baking paper and add the pistachios.
Place a saucepan over medium heat and add the caster sugar and water.

Continued

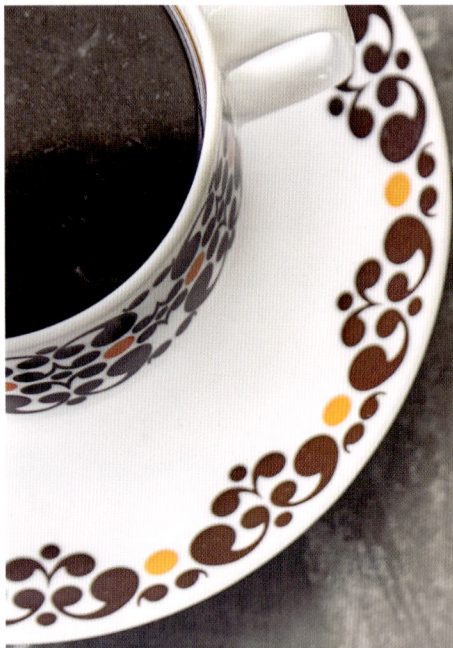

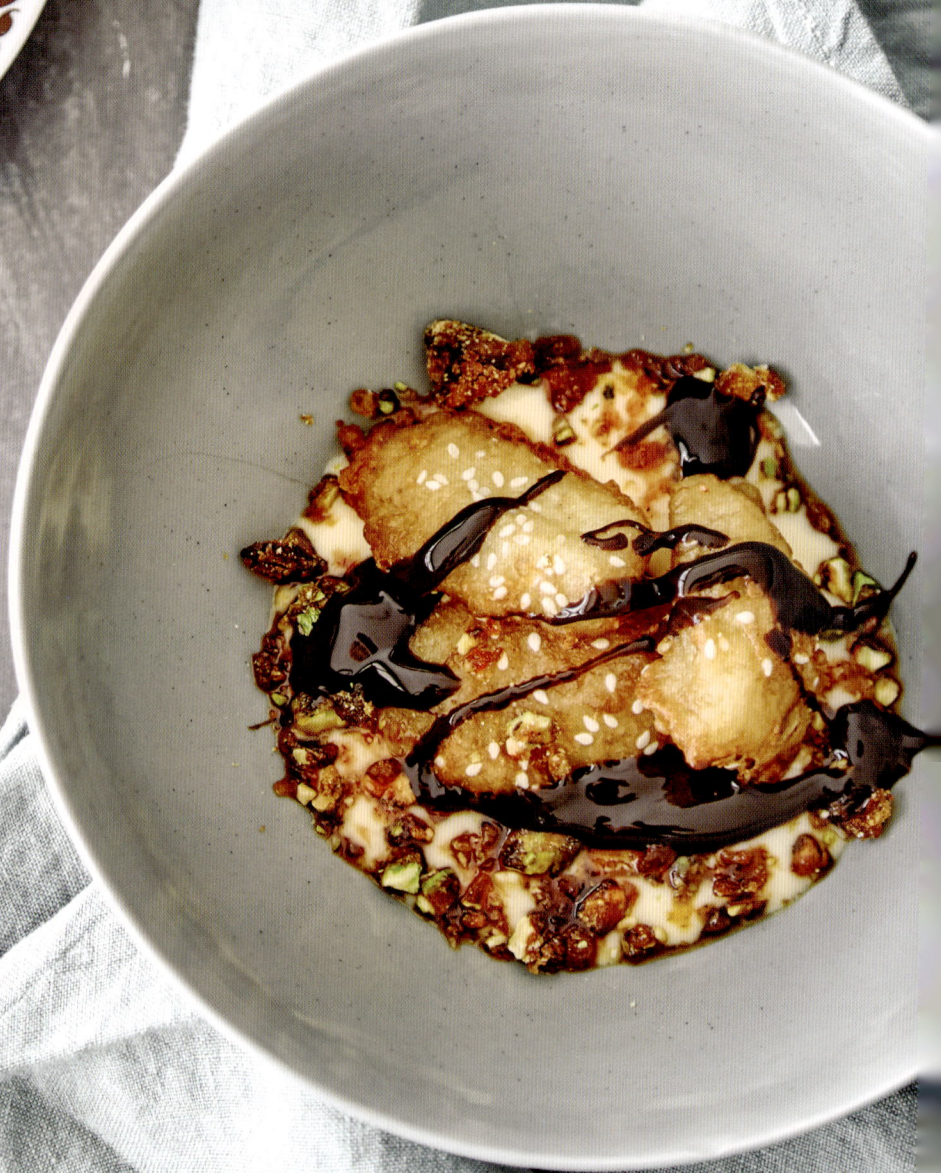

FRIED BANANA PUDDING WITH PISTACHIO BRITTLE CONTINUED...

Gently stir the sugar until it turns a deep amber gold and remove from the heat. Pour the sugar mixture over the pistachios on the baking paper, smoothing it out so it's spread evenly. Sprinkle sea salt over the brittle and set aside to cool for 15–20 minutes. When cool, shatter into small pieces with the back of a spoon and set aside in the fridge.

For the banana pudding place a saucepan over low heat and pour in the milk and cream. As the milk warms, add the cinnamon, brown sugar, golden syrup and vanilla extract and combine until the sugar and syrup have dissolved. Remove from the heat.

Add the 3 bananas to a blender. Pour over half over the milk mixture, add the cornflour and purée until smooth. Pour the banana mix back into the saucepan with the milk and place over low heat, stirring constantly and reducing by one quarter until the mixture is a thick custard. Remove from the heat and set aside to cool.

To make the fried bananas place the flour, a pinch of salt and baking soda in a mixing bowl and mix together well. Add the soda water and roughly mix the flour, ensuring the ingredients are combined but still lumpy.

Cut the 2 bananas into 12 pieces and place into a bowl. Dust the banana pieces with a little flour from the bag, then dunk them into the batter coating well.

Place a saucepan over medium heat and add the vegetable oil, ensuring it does not fill past halfway. Preheat the oven to 180°C (350°F/Gas 4).

Carefully add the battered banana to the oil and cook until golden brown, turning carefully to ensure an even color. Remove from the oil and drain on paper towels.

Place the saucepan with the pudding mixture over low heat and reheat, stirring to break up any lumps.

To serve, add the fried banana fritters to a bowl and top with a few spoonfuls of the banana pudding, then garnish with some shards of the pistachio brittle.

From The Wise

While it's okay to eat store-bought ice cream, the homemade stuff is a big no-no during pregnancy. Luckily frozen yoghurt is a delicious substitute so you can still make crazy concoctions to go with all of your homemade pies and desserts. These recipes work best if you have an ice cream machine to churn the mixture while it is freezing but if you don't have one you can always place the yoghurt mix in the freezer and stir every 20 minutes while it is setting.

PLUM & CHERRY FROZEN YOGHURT

Makes 1 litre (35 fl oz)
Cooking Time: 1 hour 50 minutes plus 4 hours to freeze.

INGREDIENTS

- × 200 g (7 oz) cherries
- × 200 g (7 oz) plums
- × 3 tablespoons golden syrup
- × 500ml (17 fl oz) Greek yoghurt
- × pinch of salt

METHOD

De-stem and pit the cherries then place them in a saucepan. Peel and pit the plums and add them to the saucepan. Pour in 125 ml (4 fl oz) water, add the golden syrup, then place the saucepan over low heat.

Bring the saucepan to the boil and drop to a simmer. Cook for 15 minutes stirring frequently. Remove from the heat and set aside in a bowl to cool in the fridge for 1 hour or so.

Pour the plum cherry mix into a blender along with the Greek yoghurt and salt. Pulse mixture until well combined.

Set up your ice cream machine as per the manufacturer's instructions and churn, then place in the freezer for 4 hours before serving.

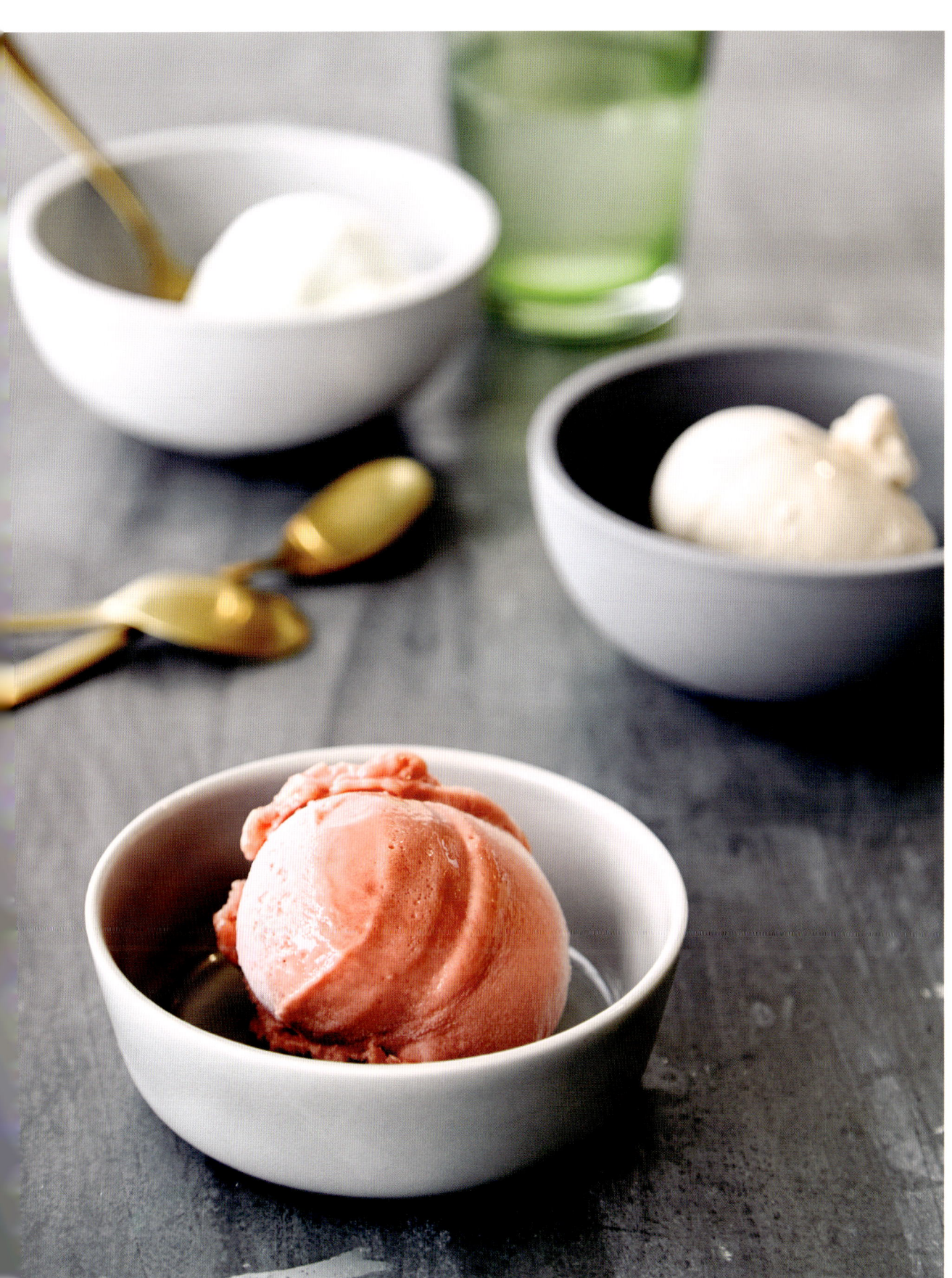

COCONUT, DATE & MOLASSES FROZEN YOGHURT

Makes 1 litre (35 fl oz)
Cooking Time: Overnight plus 35 minutes plus 4 hours to freeze.

INGREDIENTS

- 155 g (5½ oz) dried pitted dates, roughly chopped
- 250 ml (9 fl oz) coconut milk
- 4 tablespoons desiccated coconut
- 500 ml (17 fl oz) Greek yoghurt
- 2 tablespoons molasses
- pinch of salt

METHOD

The night before: place the dates in an airtight container and cover with the coconut milk.

Set aside in the fridge overnight (or for at least 4 hours if you forget to do this step the night before).

The next day: place a dry frying pan over medium heat and add the shredded coconut and toast until it colours.

Add the dates and coconut milk, Greek yoghurt, molasses and salt to a blender and pulse until the dates are chopped into small pieces. Add the shredded coconut and pulse again.

Set up your ice cream machine as per the manufacturer's instructions and churn, then place in the freezer for 4 hours before serving.

BLUEBERRY & MAPLE SYRUP FROZEN YOGHURT

Makes 1 litre (35 fl oz)
Cooking Time: 1 hour 50 minutes plus 4 hours to freeze.

INGREDIENTS

- × 200 g (7 oz) blueberries
- × 3 tablespoons maple syrup
- × 3 bananas
- × 500 ml (17 fl oz) Greek-style yoghurt
- × pinch of salt

METHOD

Place the blueberries in a saucepan, add 75 ml (2 fl oz) water and the maple syrup. Place the saucepan over low heat and bring to the boil. Reduce to a simmer and cook for 10 minutes stirring frequently. Remove from the heat and set aside in a bowl to cool in the fridge for 1 hour or so.

Add the blueberry mix, bananas, Greek yoghurt and salt to a blender. Pulse mixture until well combined.

Set up your ice cream machine as per the manufacturer's instructions and churn, then place in the freezer for 4 hours before serving.

Funtastic Baby Facts

Did you know 70 percent of newborns are born with stork bites, angel kisses, salmon patches and vascular stains? These normally fade within a few months.

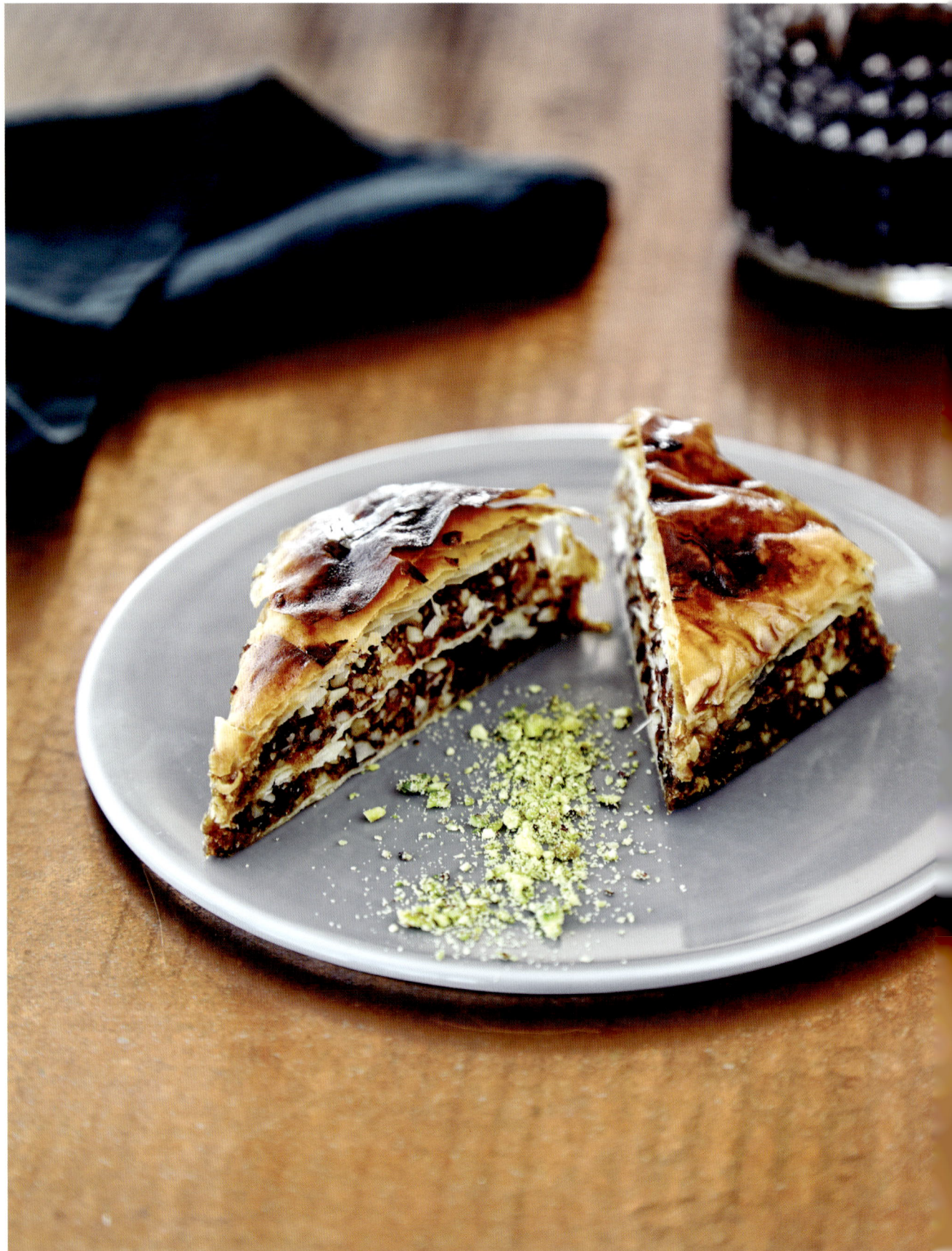

DATE & MACADAMIA BAKLAVA

Makes 24
Cooking Time: 55 minutes

INGREDIENTS

BAKLAVA

× 170 g (6 oz) dried dates, finely sliced

× 175 g (6 oz) macadamia nuts

× 1 teaspoon ground cinnamon

× 2 tablespoons caster (superfine) sugar

× 250 g (9 oz) unsalted butter, plus extra for greasing the baking tray

× 375 g (13 oz) packet of filo sheets

MOLASSES GLAZE

× 125 g (4½ oz) caster (superfine) sugar

× 3 tablespoons molasses

× 1 lemon zest

METHOD

Preheat the oven to 180°C (350°F/Gas 4). Grease a 25 cm x 30 cm (10 in x 12 in) baking tray with some butter. Place the dates in a mixing bowl.

Place the macadamia nuts in a food processor and pulse several times, breaking them into a crumble, then add to the mixing bowl.

Add the cinnamon and caster sugar and mix together well, set aside.

Place the butter into a small saucepan over low heat and melt, then remove from the heat.

Divide the filo pastry sheets into three piles.

Take the first pile and one by one brush each sheet with the melted butter, then lay the filo pastry on the baking tray. When you have used the first third of the filo, spread half the date/nut mixture evenly across the pastry. Repeat the process with the second pile of filo then spread the remaining date/nut mixture to evenly cover the pastry. Layer and butter the last third of the filo over the top then use a sharp knife to cut the pastry into squares, trimming off any excess. Bake in the oven for 25 minutes.

To make the molasses glaze, place a saucepan over medium heat and add the caster sugar, molasses, 250 ml (9 fl oz) water and lemon zest. Stir well, making sure the liquid is combined and bring to the boil, dropping to a simmer and reducing by a third.

Remove from the heat and remove the lemon zest, then pour into a heatproof container and refrigerate until needed.

Remove the baklava from the oven and spoon half the molasses glaze over the top of the pastry. Wait 10 minutes to cool and spoon the rest of the glaze over the top.

This dish is a pretty simple one to put together if you have been clever enough to make the date & coconut frozen yoghurt and are looking for some different things to do with the leftovers (if not, it goes well with some simple store-bought vanilla ice-cream).

GLAZED PEACHES WITH DATE & COCONUT FROZEN YOGHURT AND BURNT NUT CRUMBLE

Serves 4
Cooking Time: 15 mins

INGREDIENTS

- × 4 peaches
- × juice of 1/2 a lime
- × pinch of sea salt
- × 2 tablespoons unsalted butter
- × 2 tablespoons golden syrup or honey
- × 2 tablespoons apple cider vinegar
- × 8 tablespoons date & coconut frozen yoghurt (see page 196)
- × 4 tablespoons burnt nut crumble (see page 64)

METHOD

Cut the peaches in half and remove the pits, then slice into 2 cm (½ in) thick pieces. Add the peaches to a mixing bowl and squeeze over the lime and a pinch of salt. Set aside for 10 minutes.

Heat the butter in a frying pan over medium heat and add the peaches. Cook until the fruit starts to colour, then add the golden syrup. Cook the peaches until they caramelise, then flip and cook the other side. Remove from the heat and add the apple cider vinegar, swirling the fruit around in the pan.

Place the glazed peaches into a bowl and serve with a generous scoop of the coconut, date & molasses frozen yoghurt and some of the burnt nut crumble.

POPSICLES

These are a great way to make healthy and tasty little treats and they are great practice for all those upcoming kids parties and summer holidays you've got to look forward to. I've made a few different combinations but feel free to come up with your own or even try the frozen yoghurt recipes (the plum & cherry on page 194 is delicious). You will need to buy some popsicle moulds to make these, but failing that you could freeze them in some plastic cups with clean popsicle sticks or just freeze the mixture as ice cubes and put them in drinks as a bit of a surprise.

WATERMELON POPSICLES

Makes 4 (depending on the size of your mould)
Cooking Time: 10 minutes plus 3 hours to freeze

INGREDIENTS
× 450 g (1 lb) watermelon flesh, cut into chunks
× 1 tablespoon freshly squeezed lime juice
× 1 tablespoon honey
× ¼ bunch basil

METHOD
Place the watermelon in a food processor and add the lime juice and honey. Roughly tear the basil leaves and place one into each popsicle mould. Add the rest to the blender.

Blend the ingredients until there are no chunks, then pour into each popsicle mould until they are two-thirds full. Freeze for 3 hours.

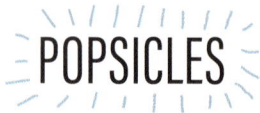

GRAPEFRUIT POPSICLES

Makes 4 (depending on the size of your mould)
Cooking Time: 20 minutes plus 3 hours to freeze

INGREDIENTS

* ½ ruby red grapefruit, peeled and deseeded
* 3 oranges, peeled and deseeded
* ¼ bunch coriander (cilantro)
* 1 tablespoon honey

METHOD

Place the grapefruit and orange in a food processor and add the coriander and honey.
Blend the ingredients until there are no chunks, then pour into each popsicle mould until they are two-thirds full. Freeze for 3 hours.

APPLE POPSICLES

Makes 4 (depending on the size of your mould)
Cooking Time: 15 minutes plus 3 hours to freeze

INGREDIENTS

* 5 green apples, peeled
* 15 g (½ oz) ginger
* 1 tablespoon lemon juice
* 1 tablespoon honey
* ¼ bunch of mint

METHOD

Place the apples and ginger in a food processor and add the lemon juice, honey and mint.
Blend the ingredients until there are no chunks, then pour into each popsicle mould until they are two-thirds full. Freeze for 3 hours.

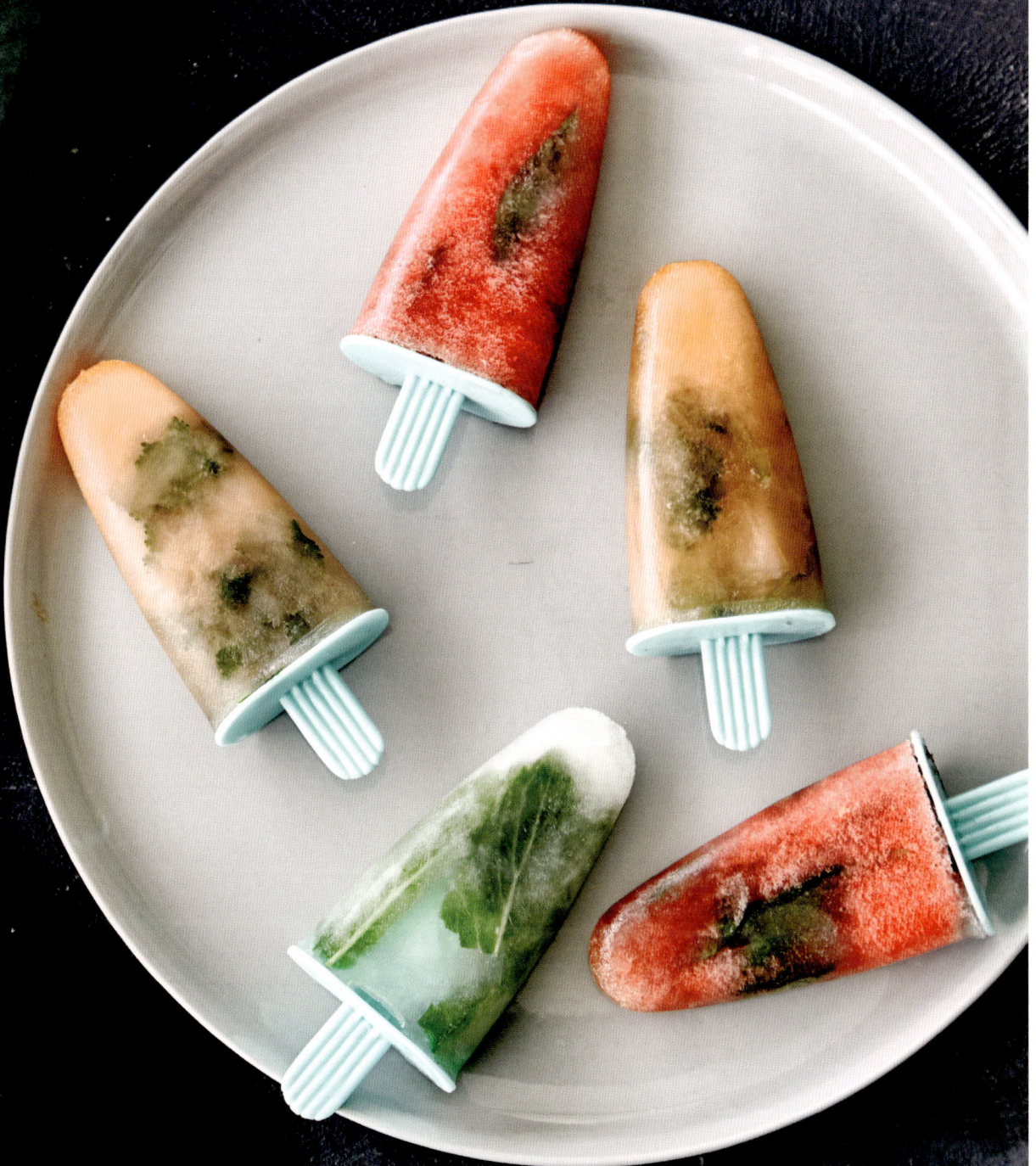

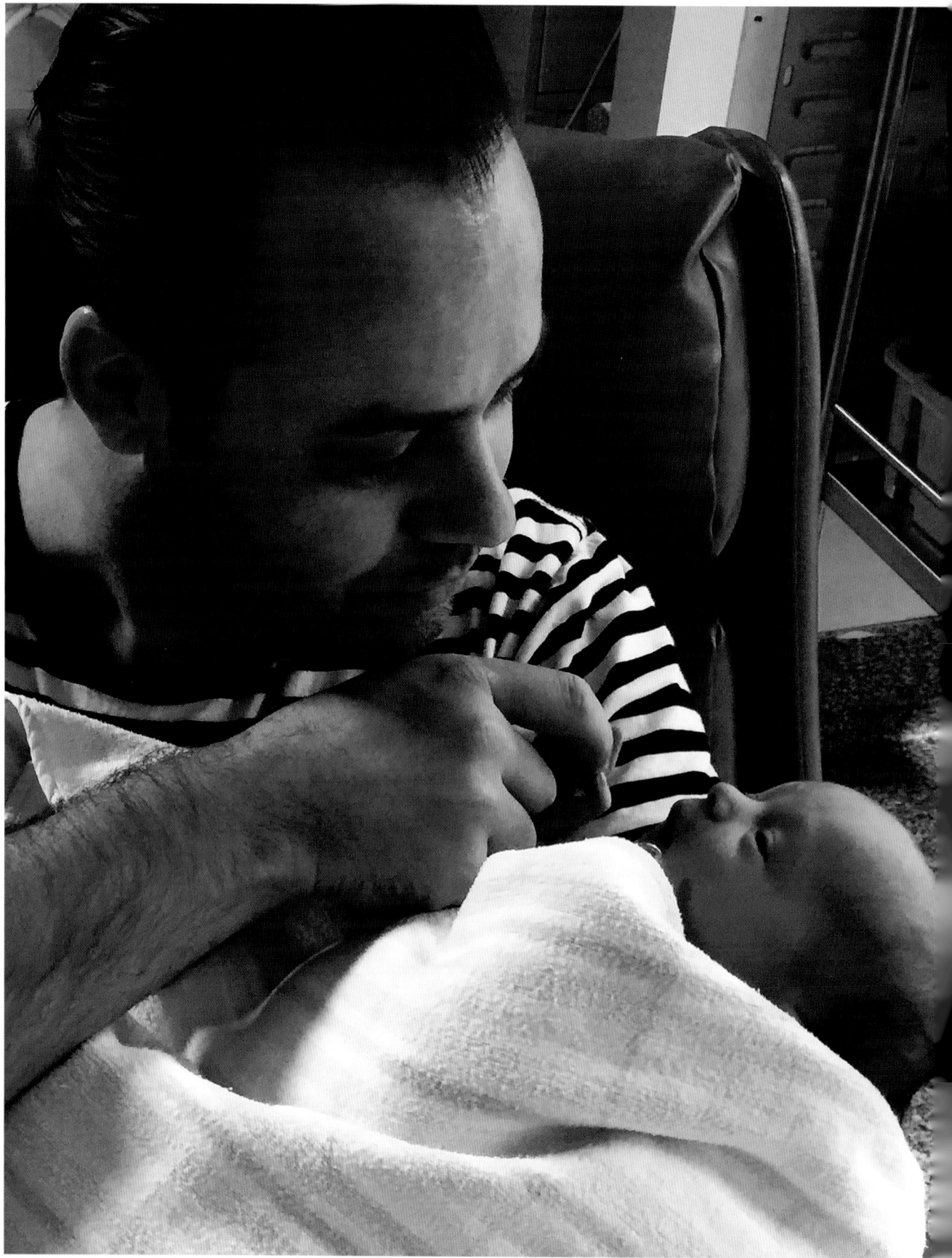

THE FIRST DAY OF THE REST OF YOUR LIFE

You never forget the day your child is born.

For some it may come out of the blue, one moment you're blissfully asleep, the next you are madly dashing to the hospital in a panic while telling your partner to breathe and be calm. Others may have to wait days or even weeks after the due date, causing you to try every remedy and old wives' tale to coax that little one out. My wife and I missed out on all that fun as we found out she had to have a caesarean section a few weeks before the due date, which unfortunately for our daughter was two days before Christmas (poor little thing never stood a chance of getting good gifts).

Aside from my daughter's birth, there are several things I will always remember about that day.

I remember waking up pre-dawn after a fitful night's sleep and driving to the hospital with *Don't Stop Believin'* by Journey playing on repeat. I remember Sam, the little boy I met as I sat next to my daughter's crib in the high dependency ward, giving out gifts to the sick babies with the money he'd saved from his allowance. I remember the cries of feeding frenzied newborns and their white knuckled parents who roamed the halls of the maternity ward like the walking dead, desperately trying to get their child to sleep. And I remember the never-ending chime of the call bell that echoed out across the ward, night and day without end as I lay sleepless on the fold out 'single bed' seemingly designed for maximum discomfort by the Marquis de Sade himself.

But above all of these memories, the one that sticks in my mind the most, is the tragic look of disappointment on my wife's face as she sat up in her hospital bed and gazed upon the food on her lunch tray. Don't get me wrong, I have nothing bad to say about hospitals, hospital staff or the food they serve (in fact if you ask me they are unsung heroes) but after going through the trauma of birth and nine months of pregnancy it's our job as partners to make sure that the first meal they get to have is something they really want, preferably containing stuff they couldn't eat before.

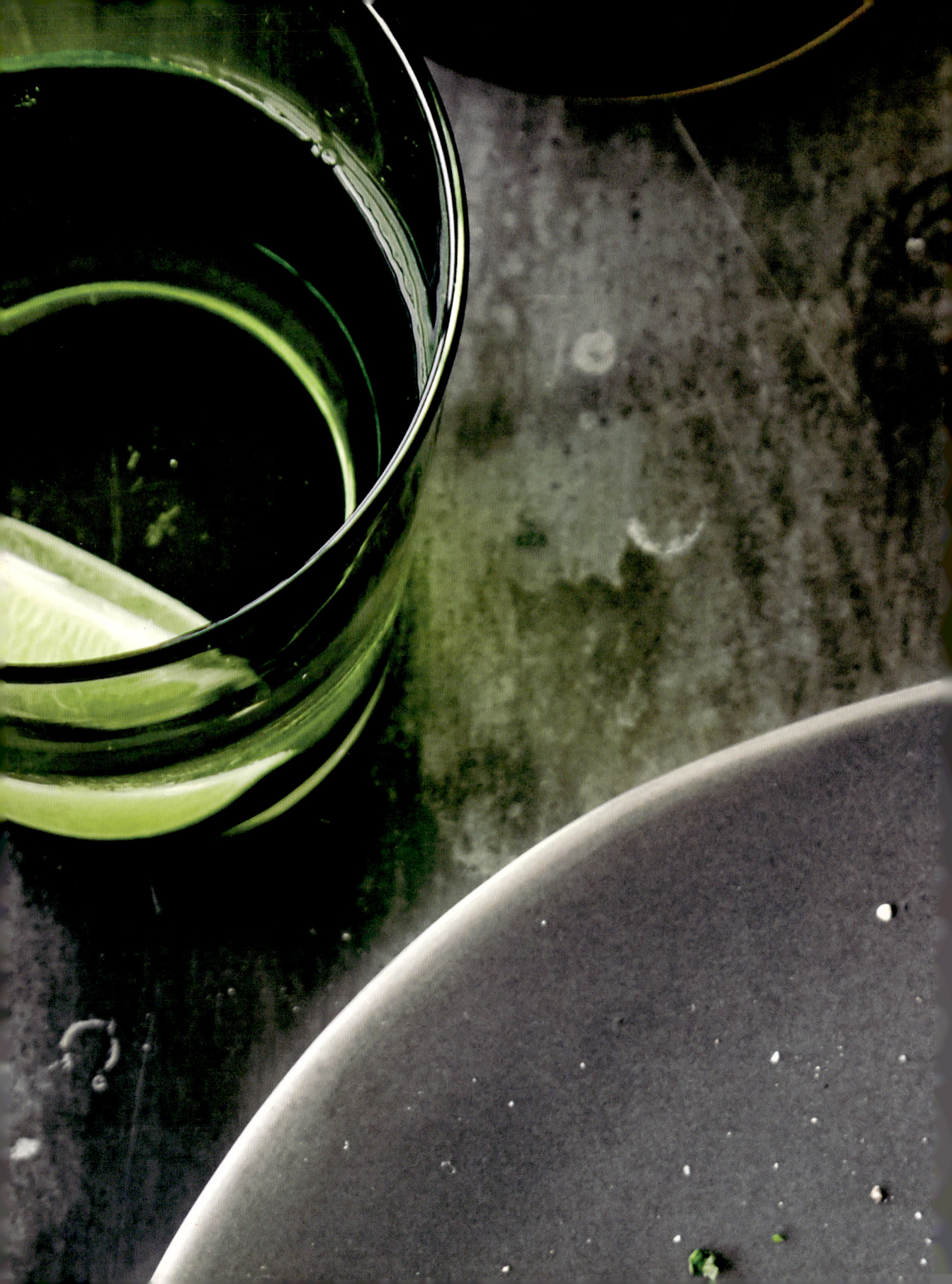

HOSPITAL FOOD

No, not what you're thinking...a couple of meals you can bring to the hospital or make when you get home featuring all the goodies that have been off limits for nine long months.

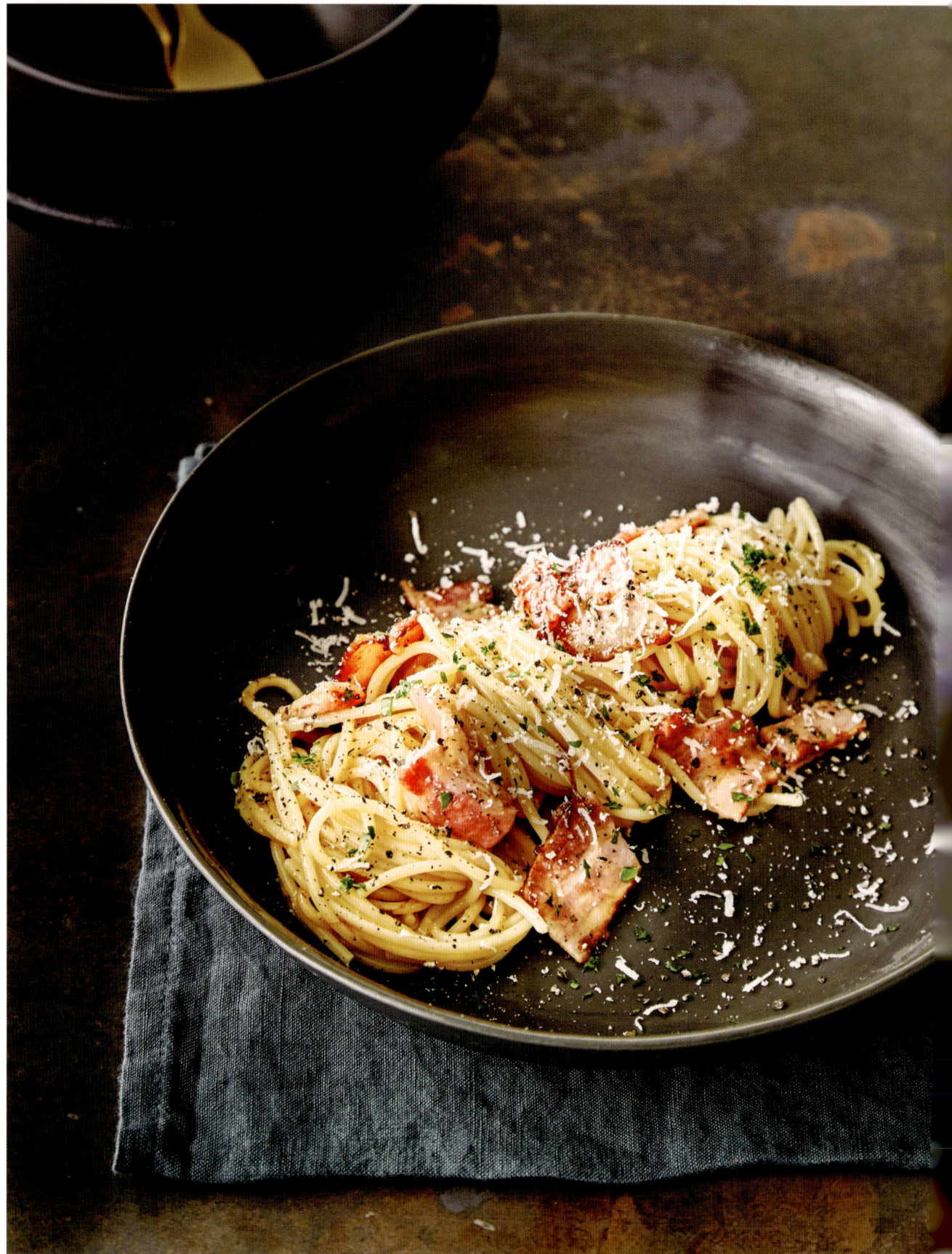

This is the first dish I made and took to the hospital for my wife after she had our little one.
The reason?
It's easy to make, is absolutely delicious and breaks the rule about fully cooked eggs (which was one of the ones my wife struggled with the most). The secret to a good carbonara is cooking the eggs with just the heat of the pasta and nothing else, thickening them into a velvety rich sauce.

SPAGHETTI CARBONARA

Serves 4
Cooking Time: 30 minutes

INGREDIENTS

- × 2 eggs
- × 2 egg yolks
- × 60 g (21/4 oz) parmesan cheese, grated plus more for garnish
- × 2 tablespoons cracked black pepper plus more for garnish
- × 6 streaky bacon slices (I prefer hickory smoked but that's up to you)
- × 2 garlic cloves, peeled
- × 400 g (14 oz) dried spaghetti

METHOD

Bring a saucepan of salted water to boil.

Put the eggs and egg yolks into a large mixing bowl. Add the parmesan cheese and 2 tablespoons of cracked black pepper to the eggs and mix together well. Set aside.

Heat some olive oil in a non-stick frying pan over medium heat. Add the bacon and garlic cloves, cooking until slightly coloured, then turn and repeat. Discard the garlic and remove the bacon from the pan. Cut into large chunks and set aside. (Do not discard the bacon fat.)

Cook pasta until *al dente* and drain.

Heat the pan with the bacon fat in it and add the bacon and the pasta, tossing well so the spaghetti has absorbed all of that wonderful bacon grease flavor.

Add the hot pasta to the bowl with the egg mixture and combine well. The heat from the pasta will cook the eggs without scrambling them. Make one of the Simple Salads (page 103-106) and transport this all back to the hospital post haste (stopping only to get a bunch of flowers). The look on your partners face when they get to eat something that has been off limits for months on end is more than worth the effort, trust me!

It's a bit unfair that a pregnant woman isn't allowed to eat stuffing unless cooked separately from the bird (which technically is not stuffing at all, it's more like stuff). Stuffing is one of life's true delights and I believe that this wonderful mash of bread, spices, meats and nuts that is lovingly mixed together and then shoved into the cavity of unsuspecting poultry should be on the menu as soon as possible after the little one has finally made their big entrance into the world. Serve with delicious duck fat potatoes.

ROAST CHICKEN STUFFED WITH PINE NUTS, GOATS CHEESE AND PROSCIUTTO

Serves 6
Cooking Time: 1 hour 55 minutes

INGREDIENTS

ROAST CHICKEN & STUFFING
- × ⅓ loaf sourdough bread, crusts removed
- × 125 ml (4 fl oz) low-fat milk
- × 2 pork sausages
- × 50 g (13/4 oz) pine nuts
- × 1 onion, finely chopped
- × 4 slices prosciutto, thinly sliced
- × 50 g (13/4 oz) goat's cheese, crumbled
- × 2 tablespoons flat-leaf (Italian) parsley, finely chopped
- × 2 tablespoons chives, finely chopped
- × 4 thyme sprigs, finely chopped

- × 1 chicken
- × 5 garlic cloves, unpeeled
- × salt and freshly ground black pepper, to season

- × duck fat, for basting

DUCK FAT POTATOES
- × 4 potatoes, peeled and roughly chopped
- × 3 thyme sprigs, leaves picked and chopped
- × 4 tablespoons duck fat
- × sea salt, to season

GRAVY
- × 5 thyme sprigs
- × 100 ml (31/2 fl oz) white wine
- × 250 ml (9 fl oz) chicken stock (see Basics, page 31 or unsalted if using store bought)
- × 50 g (13/4 oz) butter
- × 1 teaspoon plain (all-purpose) flour (optional)
- × sea salt and cracked black pepper, to season

Continued ↘

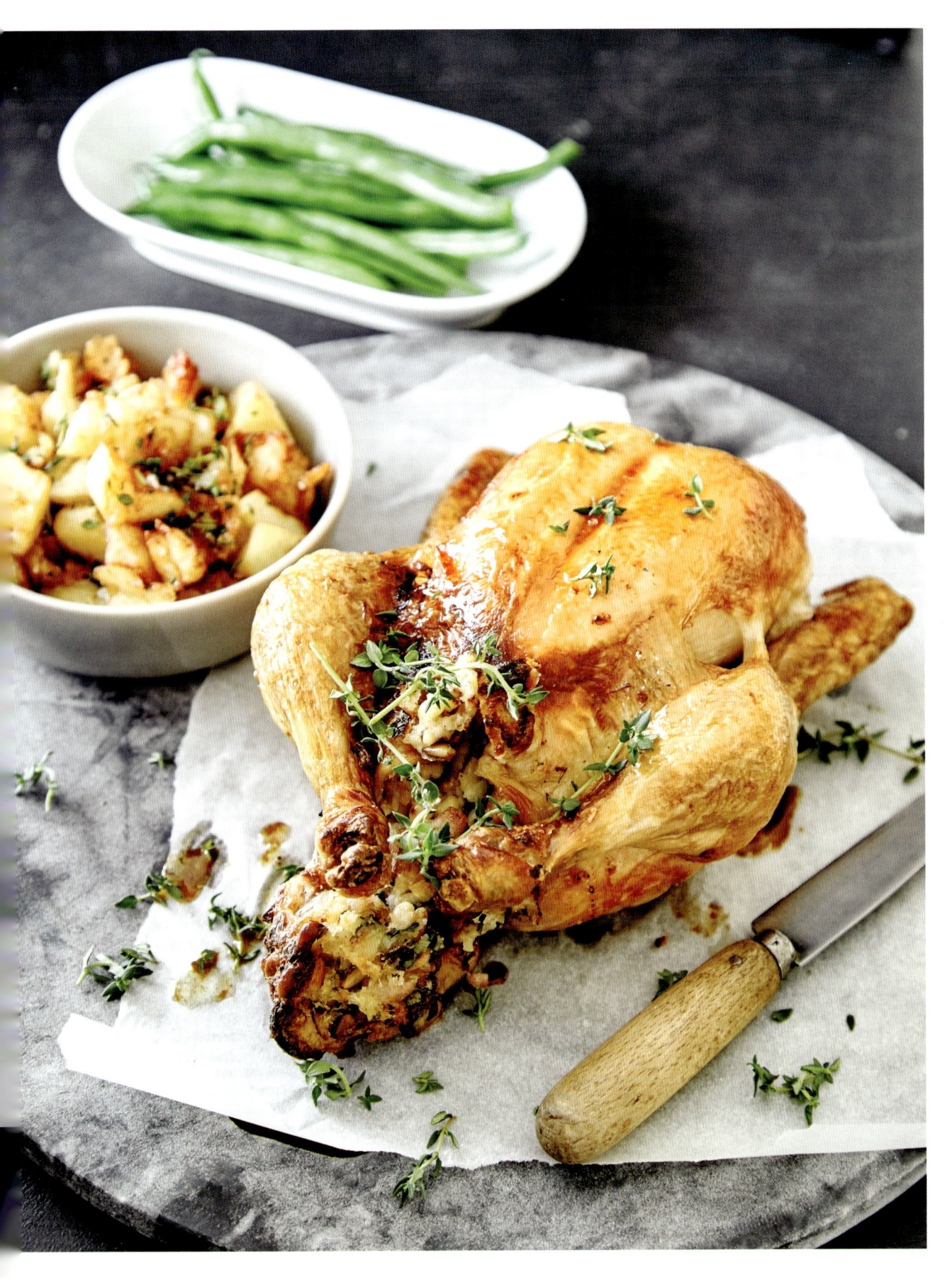

ROAST CHICKEN STUFFED WITH PINE NUTS, GOATS CHEESE AND PROSCIUTTO CONTINUED...

Preheat the oven to 200°C (400°F/Gas 6).

Tear the bread into chunks and place in the food processor. Pulse until crumbs. Place the breadcrumbs in a small bowl and add the milk. Set aside for 20 minutes.

Remove the sausages from their skins and cut the meat into small pieces.

Place a frying pan over low heat and cook the pine nuts until fragrant, then place them in a mixing bowl.

Place the same frying pan over medium heat, drizzle a little olive oil and cook the sausages, onions and prosciutto until brown. Add to the bowl with the pine nuts.

Add the breadcrumbs, goat's cheese, parsley, chives and thyme to the bowl. Season with salt and freshly ground black pepper and mix well.

Place the chicken on a baking tray and fill the cavity with the stuffing mix. Truss the chicken and baste with duck fat. Place the chicken breast side down on a wire rack in a roasting tray and scatter the garlic on the bottom of the tray. Roast in the oven for 30 minutes.

Place a pot half-filled with water over high heat and bring to boil. Carefully place the potatoes into the boiling water and cook until soft, checking if they are done by poking one with a bamboo skewer. Drain the potatoes and set aside.

Remove the chicken from the oven and carefully turn over so the breast side is facing up. Return to the oven and cook for a further 40 minutes, basting with duck fat every 10 minutes to ensure golden crispy skin.

Place a pot over medium heat and add the duck fat. When the fat is hot (test with a piece of potato, should bubble instantly), carefully add the potatoes and fry until golden on all sides.

Remove the potatoes from the heat and drain on a plate lined with paper towels and season with sea salt and thyme. Cover to keep warm.

Remove the chicken from the oven and poke the joint at the top of the thigh with a skewer to test if the bird is fully cooked, juices should run clear with no blood. Remove the chicken from roasting tray and cover with foil to rest.

Place the roasting tray that has all of the chicken juices and burnt garlic over a low flame and add the thyme sprigs. Deglaze the pan (a fancy way of saying add cold liquid to hot pan to get off all the burnt stuff) with wine and cook down the liquid by half, scraping the brown goodness off the bottom of the tray.

Place a saucepan over medium heat and pour in the roasting pan liquid, then add chicken stock. Simmer over low heat until the liquid is reduced by half. When the liquid is reduced, strain it over a bowl with a fine mesh strainer making sure you press through all of the juices.

Pour the gravy into a clean saucepan (or rinse the one it was just in) and cook over low heat, whisking in the butter (and flour if you need to thicken it a bit) and cooking until it reaches sauce consistency. Season with sea salt and freshly ground black pepper to taste and set aside.

Place the chicken on a serving platter or large board and snip the twine. Scoop out the stuffing and place in a bowl. Scatter the potatoes around the bird. Pour the gravy into a gravy boat and serve.

From The Wise

Like revenge, ceviche is a dish best served cold and after nine months of following the strict do's and don'ts of the pregnancy diet this Mexican classic should make a welcome change. The key to this dish is making sure you have very, very fresh fish, chopping the chillies and the cucumber as small as possible and slicing the garlic and radish as thin as possible.

KINGFISH CEVICHE WITH PICKLED JALAPEÑOS AND FRIED GARLIC

Serves 4
Cooking Time: 35 minutes

INGREDIENTS

- × 80ml (3 fl oz) apple cider vinegar
- × ½ tablespoon brown sugar
- × ½ tablespoon fish sauce
- × 2 jalapeño chilies, deseeded and finely diced
- × 2 radishes, finely sliced
- × 2 tablespoons olive oil, plus extra for dressing
- × 2 garlic cloves, peeled and thinly sliced

- × 400g (14 oz) kingfish filets, pin-boned and skinned
- × 1 lemon, juiced
- × 2 limes, juiced
- × 1 cucumber, deseeded and finely diced
- × ½ bunch of coriander leaves, chopped
- × 1 spring onion stalk,
- × sea salt and cracked black pepper, to season

METHOD

Add the apple cider vinegar, brown sugar and fish sauce to a container with a lid and combine well. Add the jalapeño chilies and radishes, seal the container and place in the refrigerator for 30 minutes.

Heat 2 tablespoon of the olive oil in a frying pan over medium heat. When hot, add the garlic, and fry until golden. Remove from the heat and set aside on a paper towel.

Slice the kingfish into bite size pieces and place in a bowl. Add the lemon juice and the lime juice and refrigerate for 5 minutes.

When you are ready to serve grab a large bowl add the kingfish and the pickled jalapeño chilies and radishes and drizzle one tablespoon of the pickling liquid for dressing. Add the cucumber, coriander, spring onion and season with sea salt and cracked black pepper.

Toss together well until combined. Add a drizzle of olive oil and crumble the fried garlic chips.

Serve cold.

A ham sandwich is one of life's simple pleasures that we all take for granted. But when it's taken off the menu for nine long months, it's these simple dishes that are often missed the most. This is a great snack to have on standby, it's easy to make, travels well and is absolutely delicious.

HAM, PROSCIUTTO, MOZZARELLA & PROVOLONE PANINO WITH BASIL PESTO AND ROCKET.

Serves 4
Cooking Time: 15 minutes

INGREDIENTS

- × 40g (1 ½ oz) pine nuts
- × 1 bunch of basil leaves, torn
- × 1 clove of garlic, peeled
- × 50g (2 oz) parmesan cheese, grated
- × 100ml (3 ½ fl oz) olive oil, plus extra for dressing
- × 1 ciabatta, sliced lengthways
- × 200g (7 oz) buffalo mozzarella

- × 200g (7 oz) good quality ham, thinly sliced
- × 200g (7 oz) provolone
- × 200g (7 oz) prosciutto, thinly sliced
- × 150g (5 oz) rocket leaves
- × ½ bunch basil leaves, roughly torn
- × sea salt and cracked black pepper, to season

METHOD

Grab a food processor and add the pine nuts, basil, garlic and parmesan. Blitz until there are no big chunks, then with the motor running add the olive oil in a thin steady stream until the oil is incorporated and the ingredients form a paste.

Place the ciabatta on a chopping board and drizzle some olive oil over the top and bottom.

Liberally spread the pesto over one side of the ciabatta then top with mozzarella, ham, provolone and prosciutto. Close the sandwich.

Place the rocket into a bowl, dress with a drizzle of olive oil, season with salt and pepper and toss together well.

Heat up a griddle pan or sandwich press and the sandwich toast until golden and crunchy on both sides. Remove from heat and take the top off the sandwich, add the rocket and place the lid back on.

Cut into 4 pieces and serve.

This dish should be the dish you make when you are finally home from the hospital, your baby has gone to sleep and you want to treat your partner to the first steak she has eaten that hasn't been cooked to well-done in nine long months. I have made this steak rare but if that isn't quite your thing, you can cook them for 3–4 minutes longer in the oven. The results will vary also on the thickness of the steaks.

STEAK N' EGGS

Serves 4
Preparation & Cooking Time: 30 minutes

INGREDIENTS

- × 4 porterhouse steaks (nice and thick if possible)
- × 4 tablespoons sea salt
- × 4 eggs

CHIMICHURRI
- × 4 garlic cloves, roughly chopped
- × ½ bunch flat-leaf (Italian) parsley, roughly chopped
- × ½ bunch coriander (cilantro), roughly chopped

- × 125 ml (4 fl oz) vegetable oil
- × 125 ml (4 fl oz) sunflower oil
- × 100 ml (3 ⅓ fl oz) white wine vinegar
- × 3 tablespoons dried oregano
- × 1 teaspoon dried chilli flakes
- × 1 tablespoon lemon juice
- × 1 teaspoon sea salt
- × 1 teaspoon cracked black pepper

METHOD

Preheat the oven to 180°C (350°F/Gas 4).

Grab the steaks from the fridge and season both sides with sea salt and set aside (steaks should be room temperature when they hit the pan).

Place the garlic, parsley, coriander, vegetable oil, sunflower oil, white wine vinegar, dried oregano, dried chilli flakes, lemon juice, sea salt and cracked black pepper into a food processor. Cover with the lid and blend the ingredients in the processor until the mixture is combined (if there are big chunks stop the machine and scrape down the sides with a plastic spatula then continue).

Pour the chimichurri into an airtight container and set aside (it should keep in the fridge for about two weeks).

Place a saucepan of water over medium heat and bring to the boil. Add the eggs and cook for 6 minutes. Remove and place in a bowl of cold water.

Heat some olive oil in a large cast iron pan or ovenproof pan over medium heat until it is very hot.

(Continued ↘)

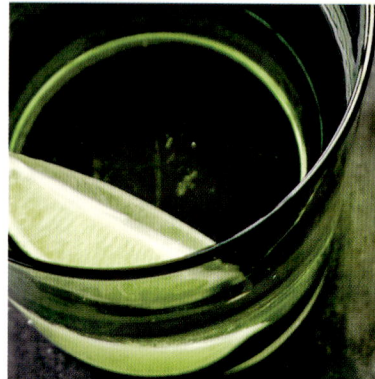

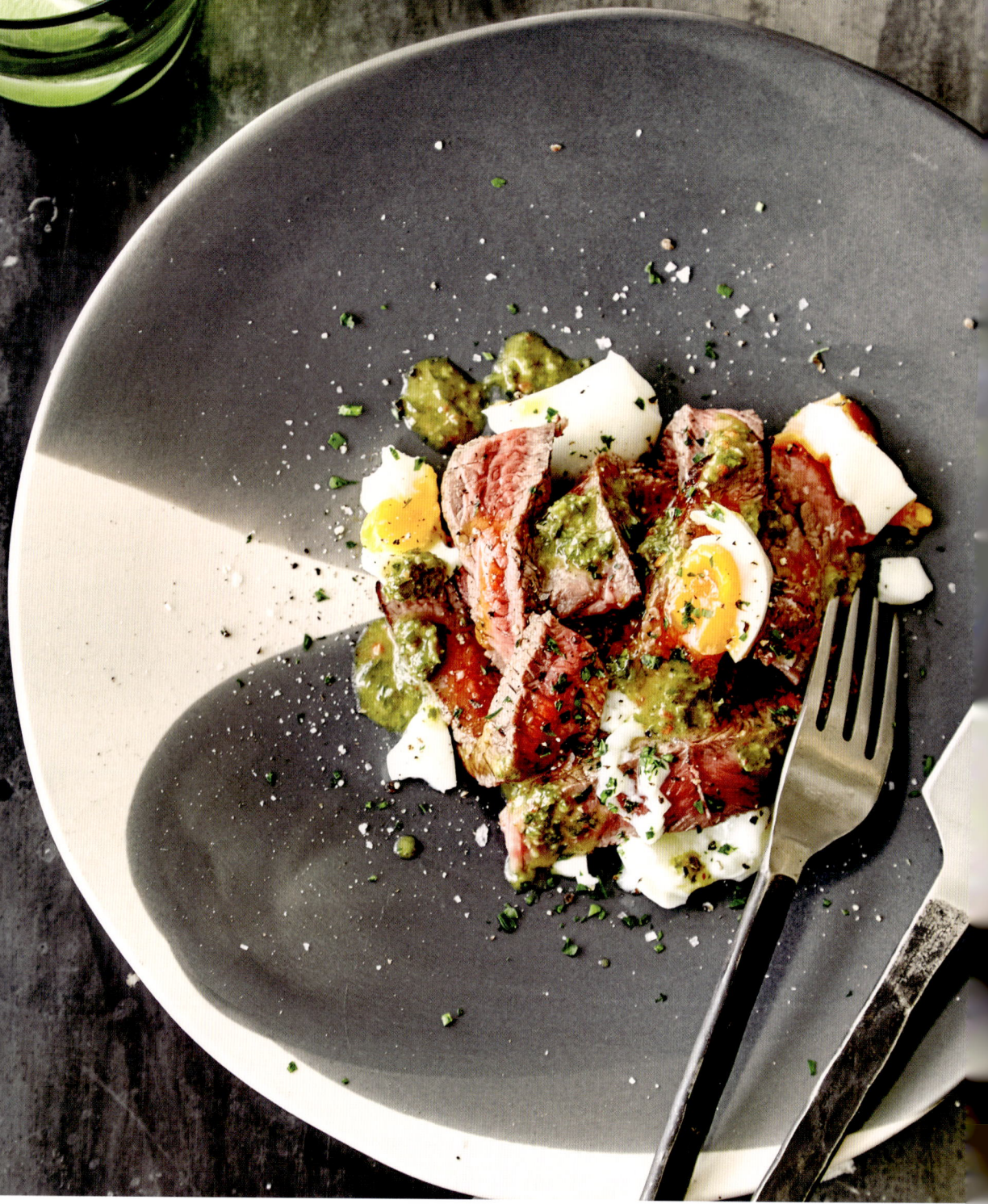

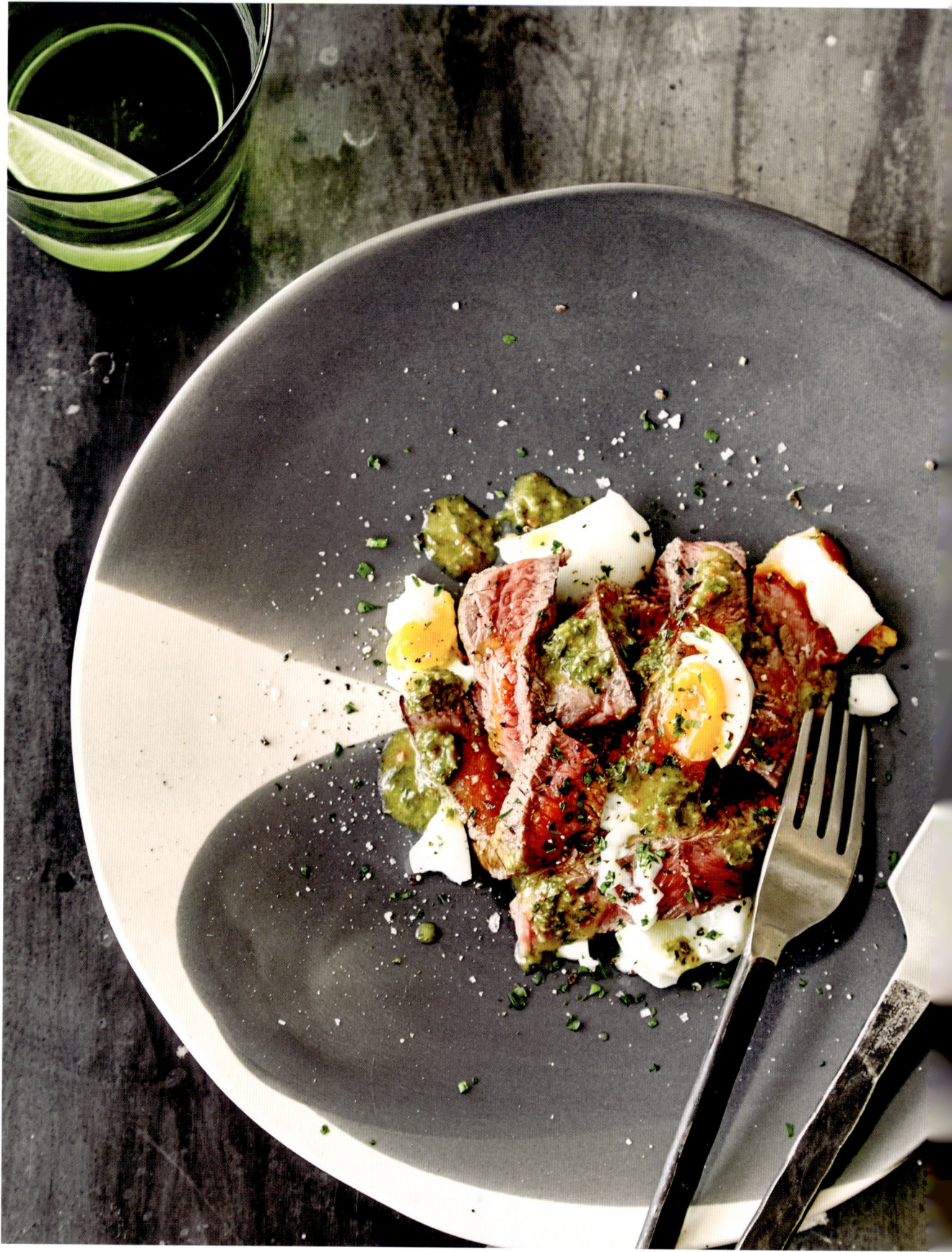

STEAK N' EGGS CONTINUED...

Add the steaks to the pan and cook for 2 minutes on one side, then flip and cook for a further 2 minutes.
  Remove the pan from the heat and place in the oven for a further 2 minutes. Carefully remove the pan from
  the oven.
Place the steaks on a chopping board to rest for 4 minutes. Peel the eggs.
Slice the steaks thinly and place on plates. Roughly break up an egg over the top of each one. Top with a few
  tablespoons of chimichurri and serve with one of the Simple Salads (page 103-106).

If you are looking for a delicious pasta to make when your home from the hospital that is easy to put together and breaks the pregnancy dietary rules, then you don't have to look much further than this. The oozing, runny goodness of burrata cheese in this dish elevates this simple pasta to another level so don't be surprised if you find yourself going back for seconds or even thirds, it's just that good.

SPAGHETTI WITH BURRATA, TOMATO AND BASIL

Serves 4
Preparation & Cooking Time: 30 minutes

INGREDIENTS

- × 2 tablespoons olive oil, plus extra for frying
- × 2 cloves of garlic, peeled and finely diced
- × 2 x 400g (15 oz) cans whole peeled tomatoes
- × 400g (15 oz) spaghetti
- × 200g (7 oz) burrata
- × ½ bunch basil leaves, roughly torn
- × ½ lemon, juiced
- × sea salt and cracked black pepper, to season
- × 40g (1 ½ oz) parmesan cheese, grated

METHOD

Fill a pot with water, add some salt and bring to a rolling boil (water should be a salty as the Mediterranean, not the Dead Sea).

Place the tomatoes into a bowl and break them up roughly with a potato masher.

Heat some olive oil in a non-stick frying pan over medium heat. Add the garlic cloves, cooking until slightly coloured, then add the tomatoes. Bring to boil then drop to a simmer for 15 minutes.

Cook pasta until *al dente*, drain (save a couple of tablespoons of the starchy pasta water).

Add the pasta water to the sauce, season with sea salt and cracked black pepper then add the pasta to the pan, toss together well then remove from heat.

Place the burrata in a bowl and break it apart roughly. Add half the cheese (as well as the cream and cheese curd that has oozed out) to the pasta and mix together well.

Place the pasta in a large serving bowl and top with the rest of the burrata, torn basil leaves, lemon juice, 2 tablespoons olive oil and a couple of extra cracks of black pepper.

Serve while hot with a generous amount of parmesan cheese and a Simple Salad (page 103-106).

ACKNOWLEDGEMENTS

To my ladies, my incredible wife Natalie and our amazing daughter Isabella. I am so blessed and so lucky to have you both in my life, this book is for you.

To my wonderful mother April. I would not have gotten this finished without all of your tireless testing, babysitting, help and support. Thank you.

To my father Thomas, thanks for teaching me how to cook, for all your recipes, testing and advice. Thank you.

To Kim, thanks for the soup inspiration and for putting up with leftovers every week while you were abandoned.

To Jeff and Lorraine, you broke the mould when you bought Natalie into the world. Thanks for letting me be part of the family.

To Vicki, thanks for the countless, selfless hours you have spent helping me. Always appreciated and never taken for granted.

To Monique, thanks for the belief, support, the dish washing and everything else you have done for me. I could not ask for more!

To Fiona, James and the team at New Holland Publishing, thank you for giving me a chance and making one of my lifelong dreams come true. I am forever in your debt.

To Ben Lee thanks for advice, really appreciate your time.

To Sue and Imogene, what an amazing couple of days! Never worked so hard, been so tired and felt so good. You are both incredible to work with, thank you both so very much.

To Andrew Quinlan and everyone who helped in the making of this book, thank you from the bottom of my heart.

Thanks to every chef who has cooked me a meal or written a book I have read, directly or indirectly you have helped create everything in here.

HOSPITAL FOOD

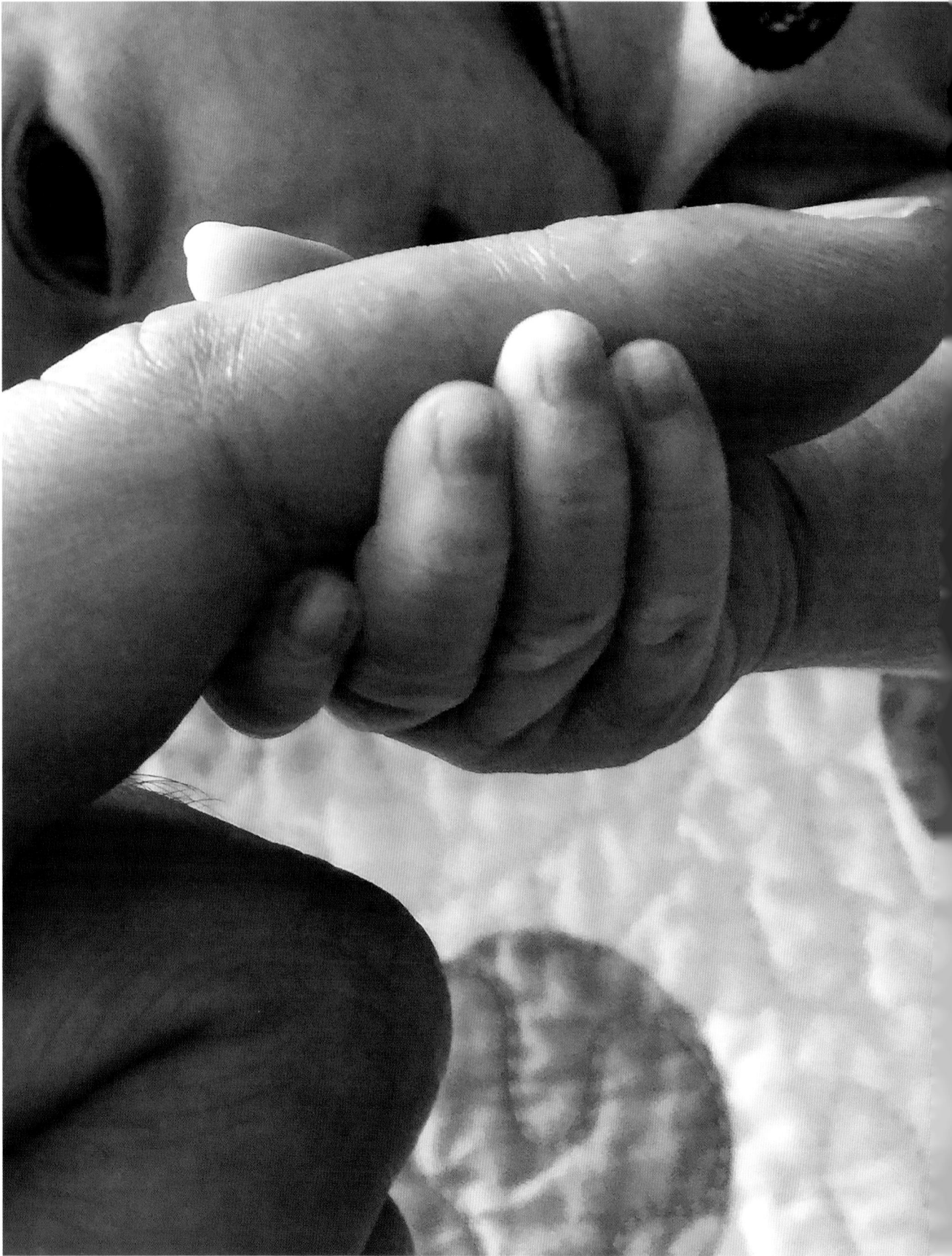

RESOURCES

Food Safety During Pregnancy.
© State of New South Wales through the NSW Food Authority.

Guidelines of Food Service to Venerable Persons.
© State of New South Wales through the NSW Food Authority.

Listeria and Pregnancy.
© State of New South Wales through the NSW Food Authority.

Salmonellosis Fact Sheet.
NSW Ministry of Health © 2016.

Having a Baby.
NSW Ministry of Health © 2016.

Folate Content of Asian Vegetables.
by Avis Houlihan, Matthew Pyke, Pieter Scheelings, Glenn Graham,
Geoffrey Eaglesham, Tim O'Hare, Lung Wong, Prapasri Puwastien and Wasinee Jongjitsin. Report Commissioned
by the Rural Industries Research and Development Corporation (RIRDC).

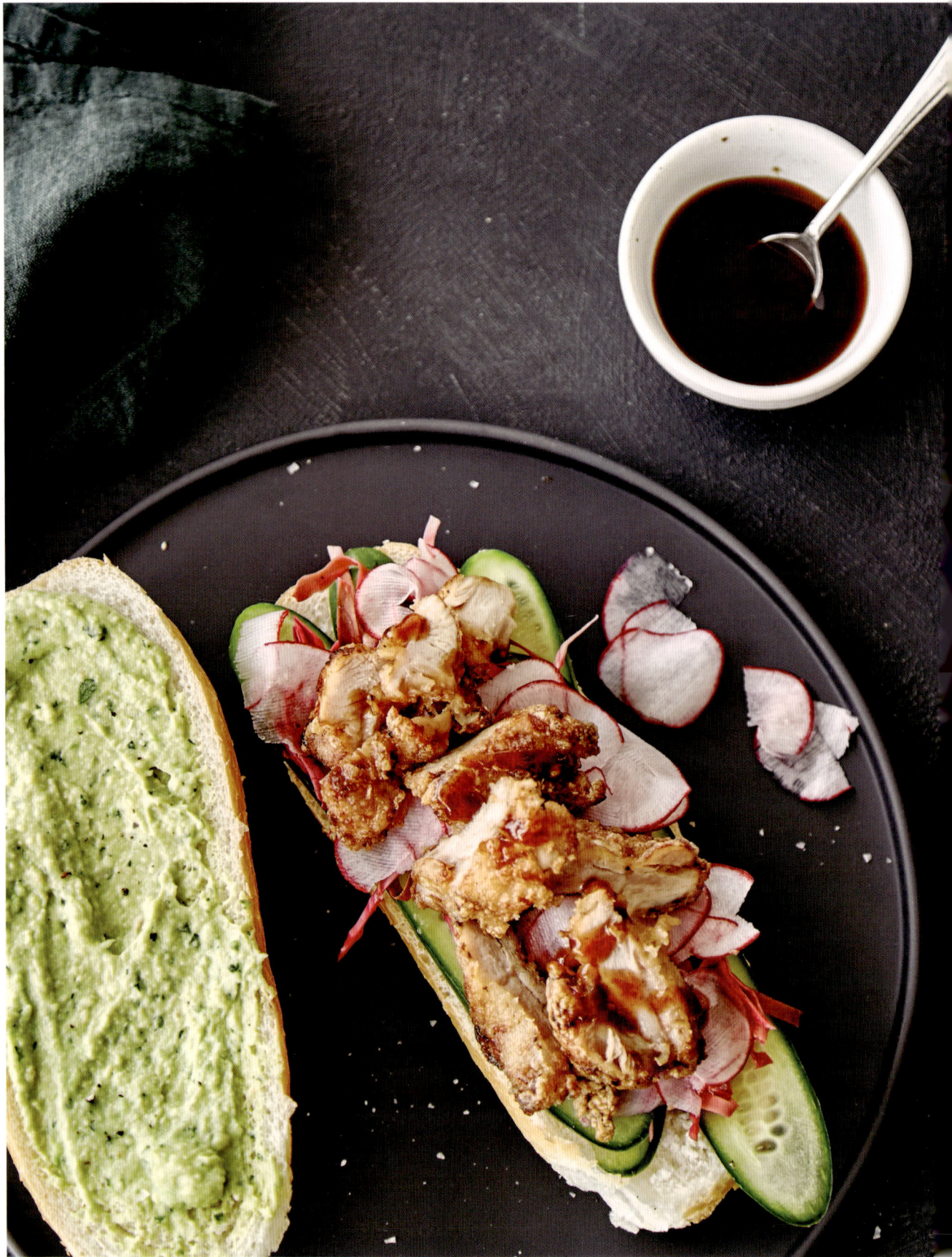

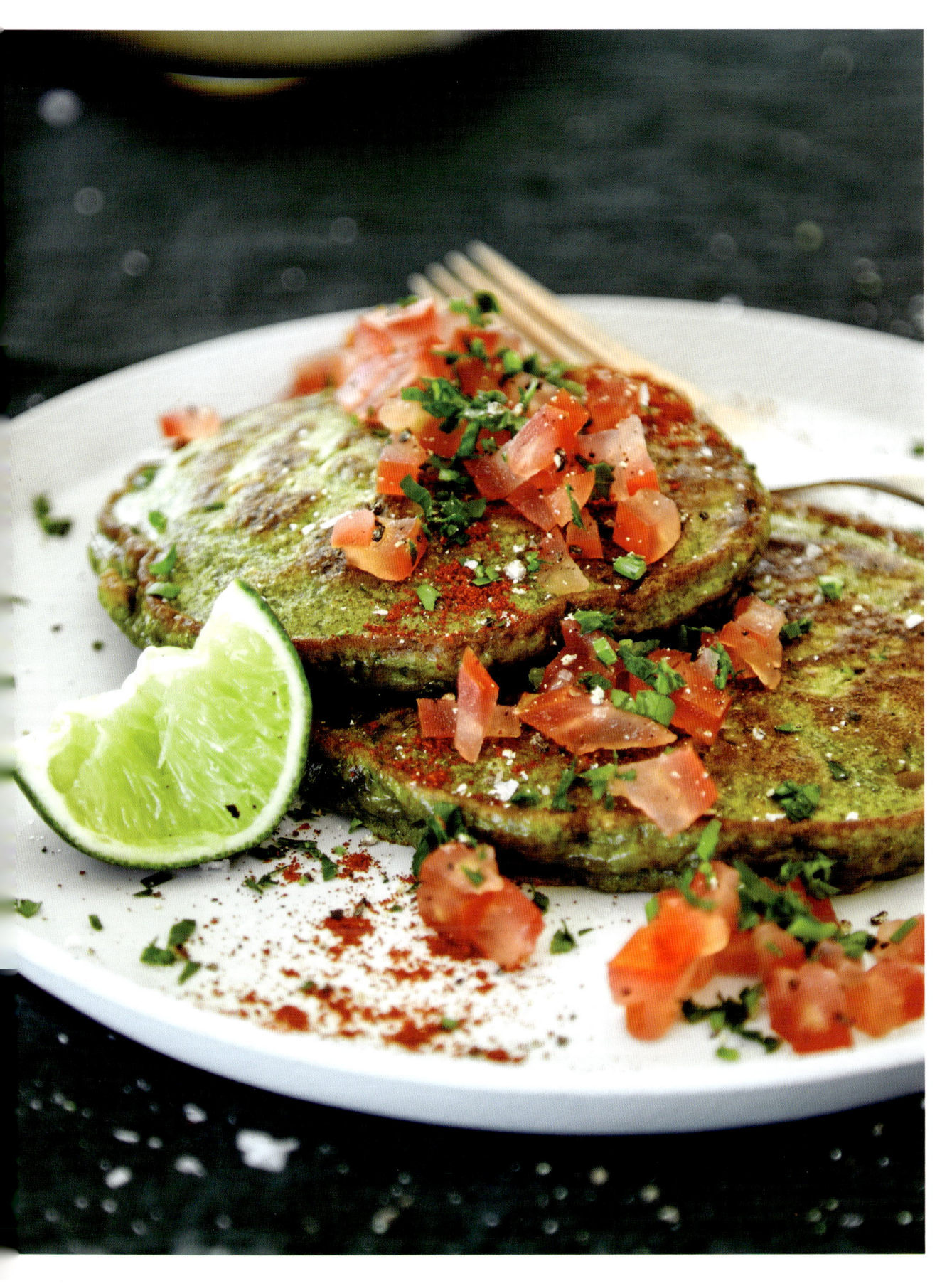

First published in 2017 by New Holland Publishers
London · Sydney · Auckland

The Chandlery 50 Westminster Bridge Road London SE1 7QY United Kingdom
1/66 Gibbes Street Chatswood NSW 2067 Australia
5/39 Woodside Ave Northcote, Auckland 0627 New Zealand

www.newhollandpublishers.com

A record of this book is held at the British Library and the National Library of Australia.

ISBN: 9781742579320
Group Managing Director: Fiona Schultz
Publisher: Monique Butterworth
Project Editor: Gordana Trifunovic
Designer: Andrew Quinlan
Photographer: Sue Stubbs
Stylist: Imogene Roache
Production Director: James Mills-Hicks
Printer: Hang Tai Printing Company Limited
10 9 8 7 6 5 4 3 2 1

Keep up with New Holland Publishers on Facebook
www.facebook.com/NewHollandPublishers

You can follow us on Instagram @theHouseHusbandsGuide or Twitter @househubbyguide